THE I

OF

HOMŒOPATHIC THEORY, PRACTICE, MATERIA MEDICA, DOSAGE
AND
PHARMACY.

COMPILED AND ARRANGED FROM HOMŒOPATHIC TEXT BOOKS
FOR THE INFORMATION OF ALL ENQUIRERS INTO
HOMŒOPATHY.

BY
DRS. F. A. BOERICKE AND E. P. ANSHUTZ.

THIRD, REVISED EDITION.

1914.

PREFACE TO SECOND EDITION.

This little book, judging from the way the first edition sold, seems to have filled "a long felt want." There have been some additions made to the new edition and the headings under Therapeutics and Materia Medica have been put in black letter type.

THE PUBLISHERS.

PREFACE TO THE THIRD EDITION.

We are gratified to know that there is no abatement in the demand for our little book and in consequence a third edition is asked for. The book was designed not for a "domestic practice," but to meet the steady call for a small, inexpensive work that would give the enquirer an insight into the theory, materia medica, therapeutics, pharmacy and dosage of Homœopathy, from which he could see whether it would be well for him to go deeper into the subject. Hundreds of copies have been sold to physicians of other schools of practice, and we have reason to believe that they have had their effect for the welfare of humanity. The book is necessarily elementary, but, we hope, the elements are such that on them can be built a sound structure of curative medicine. The aim has been to give, in the Therapeutics, the "keynotes" and the therapeutic range, of each drug, which will be a "memory refresher" to homœopathic physicians and a guide to all others.

December 1, 1913.

BOERICKE & ANSHUTZ.

CONTENTS.

Part   I. GENERALITIES 9
Part II. THERAPEUTICS 43
Part III. MATERIA MEDICA 120
           INDEX 217

The Elements of Homœopathic Theory, Materia Medica, Practice and Pharmacy.

PART I.

GENERALITIES.

SAMUEL HAHNEMANN.

First a word about the personality of Hahnemann. He was born at Meissen, Saxony, on April 10th, in the year 1755. He studied at Leipsic and Vienna, and took his degree at Erlangen, in 1779. He practiced medicine in several European cities, but, though fairly successful, financially, was dissatisfied with the results and finally gave it up for literary work. The list of his books, including translations made by him, covers 27 octavo pages in Bradford's *Homœopathic Bibliography.*

Chemistry owes a great deal to Hahnemann, who was very proficient in that science.

Practically all the modern and ancient languages, including Arabic, were at his command, and he made great use of this knowledge in his writings, especially in his homœopathic materia medica for which he laid this vast field under contribution.

He died in Paris, where he had an immense practice, in the year 1843, at the age of eighty-eight.

Such in brief was the man. Anyone wishing fuller particulars should procure *The Life and Letters of Dr. Samuel Hahnemann*, by T. L. Bradford, M. D., a work of 513 pages, the most complete life of Hahnemann, and, incidentally, history of Homœopathy, ever published.

ORIGIN OF HOMŒOPATHY.

The term Homœopathy is compounded from two Greek words: *"homoios,"* meaning similar, and *"pathos,"* meaning affection. Hence our *similia*.

In the year 1780 Hahnemann was translating Cullen's *Materia Medica* from English into German. Twenty pages in that work are devoted to Peruvian bark and these greatly excited the interest of the translator, because of the fact that it was one of the few drugs that could be relied on to definitely *cure*, and he determined to ascertain the effect of the bark on his own person. Of the effects of this experiment he wrote:

"I took, by way of experiment, twice a day, four drachms of good *China*. My feet, finger ends, etc., at first became cold; I grew languid and drowsy; then my heart began to palpitate, and my pulse grew hard and small; intolerable anxiety, trembling (but without cold rigor), prostration throughout all my limbs; then pulsation in my head, redness of cheeks, thirst, and, in short, all these symptoms, which are ordinarily characteristic of intermittent fever, made their appearance, one after another, yet without the peculiar chilly, shivering rigor."

"Briefly, even these symptoms which are of regular occurrence and especially characteristic—as the stupidity of mind, the kind of rigidity in all the limbs, but, above all, the numb, disagreeable sensation, which seems to have its seat in the periosteum, over every bone in the body—all these made their appearance. This paroxysm lasted two or three hours each time, and recurred *if I repeated the dose, not otherwise.* I discontinued and was in good health."

Such was the beginning of the practice of medicine according to the rule of "similars;" the distinctive school, "Homœopathy," grew out of the fact that Hahnemann's brethren absolutely rejected this rule and, so to speak, excommunicated him for persisting in it.

That the Law of Similia (as homœopaths term it) was dimly seen before Hahnemann's time is shown by what Hippocrates wrote, pointed out by Hahnemann:

"By similar things disease is produced, and by similar things, administered to the sick, they are healed of their diseases. Thus the same thing which will produce a strangury, when it does not exist, will remove it when it does."

What Hahnemann did was to discover "what disease is produced" by the various drugs, to quote Hippocrates, or, what train of symptoms each drug would produce, which train, according to his experience with the Peruvian bark, ought to be curative, according to the rule of similars, as laid down by the old Greek physician. This he ascertained by experimenting on the human system by "provings."

PROVING DRUGS.

Believing that he had discovered the method of ascertaining the true therapeutic range of drugs, and of their *Scientific* application to the healing of the sick, Hahnemann, and a number of his friends, began proving various well-known drugs in the same manner he had adopted with Peruvian bark. Very careful records were kept of the "deviations from the normal health" caused by the drugs. Each prover kept a "day book" in which his or her individual "symptoms," those caused by the drug at the time being proved, were minutely recorded. When it was thought that enough evidence of the range, or sphere, of the drug had been obtained, these day books were given to Hahnemann, who carefully sifted the

I WANT THE LATEST.

whōle mass and arranged it into the schema which has been followed more or less ever since. The general plan of the schema was to start with the mental symptoms and follow on down with those of the brain, eyes, ears, tongue, throat, and so on to the feet. These symptoms so arranged constitute the Homœopathic Materia Medica. To these also Hahnemann added well established facts as to the action of drugs obtained from his vast reading of medical literature. It was the work of a scholar and scientist of the highest order.

The provings conducted under the auspices of Hahnemann at this period are gathered into two volumes, known as *The Materia Medica Pura*, containing a total of 1,427 pages. But this work was to the active practitioner in later years what the ponderous unabridged dictionary is to the active business man, who wants a compact dictionary, or even a "speller." So in time a host of smaller Materia Medicas have sprung up, but all of them based on the original, or on similar provings of other drugs made since.

"I WANT THE LATEST."

If the reader will reflect, that. therapeutically (and that is the all of Homœopathy, *i. e.*, the law of the therapeutics), the *China* (Peruvian bark) of to-day is the same as the *China* of

Hahnemann's time; that *Mercury, Arsenic* and *Nux vomica* are ever the same and produce the same effects, he must recognize that the Materia Medica of Hahnemann and the early homœopaths is as much the "latest" as a multiplication table published a hundred years ago is as "late" as one published yesterday.

The Materia Medica may be made fuller and the symptomatology given more in detail, but until the human body and the effects of drugs on it change, the old Materia Medica will remain practically "the latest," as it is the most accurate, for Hahnemann seems to have been peculiarly fitted for keen observation as to the nicer shades of drug effects on the human body.

China (as Peruvian bark is known to-day in Homœopathy) to-day will cure symptoms similar to those produced on Hahnemann over a century ago and will continue to do so for all time. And the same holds good of all natural drugs. *They will cure the symptoms in the sick that are similar to those that they can produce on the human body.* That is the all of Homœopathy. *"Similia similibus curantur."*

DOSAGE AND POTENCY.

This has always been a burning question among homœopaths and a matter of ridicule from others. In his early practice of Homœopathy Hahnemann gave material doses of the mother tincture, or trituration, as is demonstrated by what has come down to us—one of the few of his clinical cases recorded—known as the "washerwoman case." A poor washerwoman applied to Hahnemann for relief from her illness. A friend was present. He, Hahnemann, closely questioned her as to the origin of the illness and of its symptoms. He then gave her the mother tincture of *Bryonia* and after she had gone remarked that she would be well in a day's time, which prediction came true, as the next day she was at work again and in her usual health.

early in his practice of Homœopathy he noticed that the large doses often produced an aggravation of the disease at first, even though a cure followed. This aggravation he soon saw was due to the action of the drug given in unnecessarily large doses. He began reducing them and from this point gradually developed the "dynamization" theory.

In brief, this is: That by "potentizing" remedies their power, their "spirit-like power" for cure, is immensely developed. This is where the "infinitesimal" feature of Homœopathy came in. In these days or radium and the discovery that the atom is a gross thing when compared with its "emanating particles," millions of which represent one atom or molecule, the idea of the power of the extremely infinitesimal is regarded with more respect than it was in the past, when the largest dose a patient could endure was the practice. An "atom" was at one time considered the smallest division of an element or smallest part capable of entering into chemical combination. Now electrons are seen to be antecedent to atoms, and these electrons are also believed to be made up of matter still more subtle, as subtle as light.

Is a molecule capable of being sub-divided without losing its identity? If so, to what extent? On this point there is certainly a difference of opinion and there is an abundance of physical evidence of the existence of matter when there remains no longer any chemical or scientific proof of its existence.

The true solution of the dosage question seems to be that drugs, like patients, must be individualized. Some drugs may be given in crude form while others act best in the potencies, even in very "high" potencies. From the 3d to the 6th is probably the best for beginners with the average run of medicines. (On this point, in the part devoted to therapeutics in this book, the strength of each drug most generally accepted will be given in each case.)

In his later life Hahnemann almost uniformly gave the 30th potency, ~~especially~~ ~~in chronic cases~~.

The question is often asked as to the size and frequency of the dose. In general we may say give 10 pellets, or three tablets, four times a day. *The size and frequency of the dose is not so important as to have the remedy homœopathic to the case.* But there are the formal directions which the physician can vary as he grows in experience. Here they are:

Pellets (medium size).—Dose for adults, ten pellets; for children, five pellets; for infants, three pellets.

Liquids—Dilutions.—Pour 20 drops of the liquid medicine into a tumbler half full of clear, pure water, stir with a clean spoon and keep the tumbler well covered. Dose for adults, two teaspoonfuls; for children, one teaspoonful; for infants, one-half teaspoonful.

Triturations—Powders.—Dose for adults, as much of the powder as will cover a silver ten cent piece. For children, the same quantity as for adults; for infants, half that quantity.

Tablets (Triturations made in Tablet Form). —Dose for adults, three tablets; for children, two tablets; for infants, one tablet.

Disks—or Cones.—Dose for adults, four disks; for children, three disks; for infants, two disks.

"THE CHRONIC DISEASES."

At this point it may be well to briefly outline another point in homœopathic history that has caused much discussion and some bitterness among homœopaths.

After Hahnemann had fairly well developed his discovery anent China and many other drugs he published, in 1796, his observations in *Hufeland's Journal*, the leading German medical periodical of that time. It was entitled:

"An Essay on a New Principle for Ascertaining the Curative Powers of Drugs, with a Few Glances at Those Hitherto Employed."

This was followed by *The Organon*, in 1810. Five editions appeared, the last in 1843. This was followed, in 1811, by the *Materia Medica Pura (Reine Arzneimittellehre)*. In the stormy years that followed he was finally driven from Leipsic, in 1820, and found refuge under the protection of the Duke of Anhalt-Kœthen, where he remained for fourteen years. It was during this period that he wrote his great and much disputed work, *The Chronic Diseases*, which in the English translation covers over sixteen hundred octavo pages.

Broadly speaking, in this work he attributes the origin of all chronic cases to three "miasms," *i. e.*, psora, syphilis and sycosis. The theory occupies about 150 pages of the work and the remainder is taken up with a Materia Medica for the cure of such cases. (The theoretical part of this book has been recently published separately from the main work.) Of these three "psora" was to Hahnemann what "original sin" is to the theologians. For instance, two persons are down with a given acute disease, one has it mild, while the other is desperately ill; the cause is that the latter has the "psora" taint. Some have said that Hahnemann claimed that psora was the result of "suppressed itch," but this is an error, started by superficial readers." Of late many men have come to the conclusion that Hahnemann's "psora" and tuberculosis are identical.

The remedies introduced in this book, which is largely materia medica, or many of them, were absolutely unheard of before in medicine, such as *Graphites, Lycopodium, Natrum muriaticum, Sepia, Silicea*, yet to-day these remedies, and the others given in the book, are constantly in successful use by thousands of practicing physicians and have given relief to hundreds of thousands of patients.

In these remedies the dynamization theory seems to be borne out. *Lycopodium*, for instance, was supposed to be absolutely inert, but when thoroughly triturated and run up to the 30th potency, as Hahnemann prescribed it, there can be no doubt of its wonderful efficacy when indicated by the symptoms. The same may be said of *Natrum mur., i. e.,* table salt, *undoubtedly* a powerful remedy in the 30th potency, and of the others. Mere denial is the refuge of small minds, but many doubters have tested the 30th potency of *Natrum mur.* and have been convinced.

SYMPTOMATOLOGY.

The idea is quite prevalent among many that homœopathic physicians are mere symptom hunters, and that their practice begins and ends with this. In *The Organon* Hahnemann says that when a case first comes under observation of the physician his duty is to ascertain if there be any "removable cause" for it. When this has been effectually investigated, the origin of the disease inquired into, habits, etc., *then* come the symptoms, and these, even the most trivial, may serve as a guide to the cure of a man who presents no "removable cause" for his disease. A patient, say, is very flatulent; sits down to the table with an apparently good appetite, but a few mouthfuls of food satiate him; he feels bloated; is more or less constipated; has red sand in urine; nearly always feels worse late in the afternoon; looks sallow.

The experienced reader of symptoms would

give him *Lycopodium,* and probably make a brilliant CURE.

Another patient follows. He has piles, and says so. An examination shows them to be blind, purplish, rarely bleeding. Man says it feels as if he had a chestnut burr, a lot of sharp sticks, "up there." *Æsculus hip.*, internally, and a little of the ointment of that remedy or a suppository of it, externally, and next time he is seen that man will laud the relief given him.

Another patient contracted rheumatism from cold, damp weather. In his case the origin of the ill points to *Rhus tox.* as the remedy. And so on and on indefinitely.

In brief, the true homœopathic physician has symptomatology, plus all the other branches of medicine required by first-class colleges. And the greatest of these, for the general practitioner, is his symptomatology, or Homœopathy, by which he is able to make *cures* of cases that baffle the otherwise scientific physician. There is a marvelous power in this Homœopathy though its action is so gentle as to cause many to doubt the very evidence of their senses.

In typhoid, scarlet fever, diphtheria, croup, mumps, and many other diseases, where is the "removable cause?" Sanitation, hygiene, isolation. etc., may prevent the spread of the disease, but to one in its grip there is nothing to be done but give a remedy to shorten its course and to give relief to the patient. It is in such cases that the man who has even a very superficial knowledge of Homœopathy has a big advantage over his brethren of other schools. To illustrate how great is this advantage it may be well to give, briefly, the following historical fact:

In 1831 Asiatic cholera swept over the Austrian empire and other countries of Europe. The medical profession was powerless before this then almost unknown disease. Homœopathic physicians consulted Hahnemann, giving him as complete a description of the disease and its symptoms as was possible. He had never seen a case, but from the symptoms was able to tell accurately what medicines would most successfully combat the epidemic. The result was that under the infinitesimal doses of Homœopathy the death rate was about 6 per cent. of the cases treated, while under other treatments it ran over 50 per cent.

This demonstrates what a tremendous advantage the man who is acquainted with the symptomatology of drugs has over his fellow practitioner who does not possess this knowledge.

The same holds true in all epidemics of disease, no matter what its nature, and whether it be new or old. The man who knows the principles of *Similia Similibus Curantur* has an enormous advantage over his otherwise equally, or even far superiorly learned brother physician.

Probably still greater than symptomatology is a knowledge of the *origin* of the disease; whether fron dry, cold winds, wet cold weather, hot weather, suppressed skin diseases, sudden chilling or any other cause. When the origin is known the physician can often go direct to the curative remedy.

Homœopathy, "the science of therapeutics," a law of nature, is not the private property of any one class; it is open to all who will learn of the truth, and *anyone* can learn of the truth of *similia* by study. It is a tremendous power for any physician.

HOMŒOPATHIC BOOKS.

Assuming that the buyer of this little work may develop a further taste for the study of the science of Homœopathy, a few words on the books for such study may not be amiss.

The first book should be *The Organon of the Art of Healing*, by Hahnemann. This book does not concern itself with Materia Medica or therapeutics, but exclusively with the fundamental principles underlying the science of Homœopathy, and a comprehension of these is of the utmost importance to anyone who would seek to acquire a mastery of Homœopathy, or the science of Cure.

The *Materia Medica Pura* and *The Chronic Diseases* are the basis of homœopathic materia medica, on which nearly every other work on the subject is founded. Of course, there have been other remedies added, but these two form the foundation.

The *Encyclopædia of Pure Materia Medica*, by Dr. T. F. Allen, includes the whole of the Materia Medica of Hahnemann and also of all other provings of drugs that have been made since Hahnemann's time. It is a work of ten large volumes, a homœopathic encyclopædia of Materia Medica, but it is out of print.

After finishing the ten volumes of the *Encyclopædia* Dr. Allen condensed the gist of these into *A Hand-book of Materia Medica and Homœopathic Therapeutics*, a work of 1,165 quarto pages, containing the symptomatology of 388 drugs, and, in small type in the schema of each, the verified therapeutics of each. It is the best complete Materia Medica.

Probably the most popular work on this branch, as ten editions prove, is Cowperthwaite's *Materia Medica and Therapeutics*, "the most useful book on the subject ever published for the busy practitioner." Cowperthwaite gives only verified symptoms and outlines the therapeutic scope of each drug. It is a *practical* book.

Another *very* useful book is Pierce's *Plain Talks on Materia Medica*. It doesn't deal so much with the symptomatology as with the actual use of drugs at the bedside. It is a direct guide. *Lectures on Homœopathic Materia Medica*, by Dr. J. T. Kent, is the subject put in colloquial form. It has been pronounced to be as "fascinating as a novel," but deals with symptomatology only. *A Clinical Materia Medica*, by Dr. E. A. Farrington, is chiefly a book of comparisons and differentiation between the various remedies. *The Essentials of Homœopathic Materia Medica*, by W. A. Dewey, M. D., is one of the most popular books among beginners of the study of Homœopathy. It is written as a "quiz compend;" a question, followed by the answer, and these cover the "principles" of Homœopathy, its pharmacy and the materia medica of its leading drugs.

It may seem odd to class *Leaders in Homœopathic Therapeutics,* by Dr. E. B. Nash, among homœopathic materia medicas, but the two are really interchangeable. Dr. Nash's work has been immensely popular and deservedly so (now in its fourth edition), for it is interesting in itself—to anyone—and embodies the experience of an old physician after a lifetime of useful practice. You will make no mistake in buying this book, even though you have all the others. You get a new angle in *every* book.

Keynotes and Characteristics with Comparisons of some of the Leading Remedies of the Materia Medica, by H. C. Allen, M. D., is a very valuable work and contains the materia medica of what are known in Homœopathy as the "nosodes," *i. e.*, the potentized virus of various diseases, *Tuberculinum, Bacillinum, Syphilinum,* etc., etc., remedies that work wonders in constitutional defects. Dr. Allen later wrote a work treating entirely of the nosodes.

There are many other works, large and small, on homœopathic materia medica, as may be seen by consulting the book catalogues of homœopathic publishers (send for one and keep it handy), but the foregoing are what may be termed representative works.

Homœopathic therapeutics are the materia medica applied to named diseases. Hahnemann, and the stricter homœopaths, always frowned on treating diseases by *name—treat the patient according to his symptoms regardless of what his disease is diagnosed.* Thus, ten or more different cases of any disease may call for ten or more different remedies, although each case may be properly termed, say, "typhoid," but, as, in each instance, the individual symptoms may be different, therefore, the true homœopathic method is to "treat the patient and not the disease;" *i. e.,* be guided by the symptoms and not by the *name* of the disease. In one of the leading homœopathic books on typhoid fever, over thirty remedies are given that are indicated in the varying phases of that disease.

The big "unabridged dictionary" of therapeutics is Lilienthal's *Homœopathic Therapeutics,* a large 8vo. volume of 1,154 pages. It is to therapeutics what Allen's Hand-book is to materia medica.

The latest work on the subject of general therapeutics is *Practical Homœopathic Therapeutics,* by W. A. Dewey, M. D. It is much smaller than Lilienthal's, but is *very* helpful to all who are guided by the *name* of the disease—as must generally be the case.

Another work, a student's manual, is the *Essentials of Homœopathic Therapeutics.* A quiz compend, by Dr. W. A. Dewey, that will be found *very* useful by all beginners. In a small compass it gives the leading drugs for all diseases by *name,* as, say, for "Diarrhœa," "Typhoid," "Catarrh" and so on through the list of disease *names.*

There are many other works on the subject, as may be seen by reference to any complete homœopathic book catalogue, but the above named are perhaps the best suited to the beginner and for general practice.

The "repertory" is peculiar to homœopathic practice. It is an index of symptoms giving the name of a remedy, or remedies, having a given symptom. These are arranged in many forms, from the 1,380 big pages of Kent's *Repertory of the Homœopathic Materia Medica* down to little compact pocket-books.

There are also many special repertories as on intermittent fever, tongue, urinary organs, headache, etc., etc., etc., as may be seen by reference to homœopathic book catalogues.

The following are a few of the standard works on special subjects, by homœopathic physicians that can be relied on:

Diseases of Children.—There are a number of these, but the one by Dr. C. S. Raue is the latest and most up to date in matters of diet, care, etc., etc.

Women.—*Obstetrics,* by Dr. Henry N. Guernsey, is a very large volume, published in 1878, but reprinted many times since. Obstetric methods have advanced since then, but the book *lives* because of the *therapeutics,* which do not nor cannot change in true Homœopathic practice.

A Text-book of Gynæcology, by Dr. Jas. C. Wood, is the accepted book on the subject by our homœopathic colleges, so no more need be said of it.

Fevers.—*The Therapeutics of Fevers, Con-*

tinued, Bilious, Intermittent, Malarial, Remittent, Pernicious, Typhoid, Typhus, Septic, Yellow, Zymotic, etc., by Dr. H. C. Allen, is the chief work on the subject. It does not concern itself with diagnosis, diet, etc., etc., but it is purely homœopathic therapeutics applied to fevers. An invaluable work for those who can use it—and anyone who can read disease-symptoms ought to match them with the aid of this book.

Genito-Urinary Diseases.—The two good works on this subject are *Diseases of the Urinary Organs,* by Clifford Mitchell, M. D., and *Urological and Venereal Diseases,* by Bukk G. Carleton, M. D. Two complete works on the diagnosis, prognosis, pathology, treatment, etc., etc., of this range of disease; the authors do not confine themselves to homœopathic therapeutics exclusively, but give all the accepted treatments.

For purely homœopathic therapeutics of these diseases, etc., etc., get *Sexual Ills,* a small manual compiled from homœopathic literature.

Practice.—Homœopathic works on practice differ in no particular from other works on the same subject, save as shown by the individual views of the authors, excepting in their therapeutics. There are a number of these in homœopathic literature, the leading one, perhaps, being *A Practice of Medicine,* by H. R. Arndt,

M. D., and Jousset's *Practice* is a work of about equal size, translated from the French.

There are two works on practice, both pocket size and very handy, one, *A Practice of Medicine,* by Dr. M. A. Custis, and the other by Dr. Ch. Gatchell, *A Pocket-Book of Medical Practice.*

Veterinary.—Homœopathy has gained green laurels in the field of veterinary practice, although there is no homœopathic veterinary school. The books on this subject can be found fully described in any homœopathic book catalogue.

In conclusion, we may state that the foregoing list of books forms but a very small part of homœopathic literature.

(Perhaps an apology is due here to the reader for introducing a section that reads almost like a book catalogue, but this little work is designed to *help* beginners in Homœopathy and this must be the excuse—if one is needed.)

HOMŒOPATHIC MEDICINES.

Any drug is homœopathic to the symptoms it will cause, consequently it may be said that every drug is a homœopathic drug, if we know its symptoms. But only those which have been *proved* can be administered to the sick for the cure of disease according to the law of *similia.* Furthermore, *only those prepared as they were by the provers can be fairly used.* There is, some hold, as much difference between a fresh plant tincture, and one made from the dried drug, or fluid extracts, as there is between a fresh apple and a dried one.

For instance, *Aconite* is prepared differently under the rules of the U. S. P. from what it is for homœopathic use, and it is manifestly an unfair trial to prescribe it, or the fluid extract, on homœopathic lines. In homœopathic pharmacy the *fresh, green* plants are used for making tinctures wherever possible.

In the terms of union labor, "unfair" medicines have done more harm to Homœopathy than any other one thing—careless, or downright dishonest pharmacy, the substitution of the cheaper fluid extracts and tinctures of the old school, and of the eclectics, for the more expensive homœopathic fresh plant mother tinctures, which in these days of cut-throat competition is frequently done; these are some of the drawbacks with which Homœopathy has had to contend. Given the properly prepared medicine, and the ability to apply it to its "similar" in sickness, a cure will follow, if a cure be possible. But the prescribers must have accurate medicines.

The physician who goes about seeking the "cheapest" drugs, or lets himself be talked into buying these cheap drugs, is like the mountain climber who would buy the cheapest ropes for his perilous expedition. Or like a government that would send out an old pot-metal iron-clad against a modern nickel-steel battleship—because it was "cheaper." However all this is obvious.

MOTHER TINCTURES.

These are all designated by the Greek letter theta (θ).

There are several classes of mother tinctures which differ according to the mode of preparation. Let *Aconite* serve as an illustration of one of them. The flowering plant is gathered and then pounded to a pulp; the juice is expressed from this pulp and mixed with its equal weight of pure *grain* alcohol. This is allowed to stand for eight days and is then filtered. The filtered product is *Aconite* θ.

Wherever possible, the true homœopath prepares his tinctures from the *fresh, living plant,* the fresher the better.

The exception to this rule is in drugs like *Nux vomica, Ipecac.,* etc. *Nux vomica* is prepared by adding to one part of the finely pulverized nuts five parts, by weight, of pure grain alcohol. This is allowed to stand for eight days, being thoroughly shaken twice a day, and then filtered. The product being *Nux vomica* θ.

There are several other classes of medicine,

but it is needless to go into details concerning them here.

POTENCIES.—DILUTIONS.—ATTENUATIONS.

The strict practitioner of Homœopathy believes with Hahnemann that, by dynamization, the drug power of tinctures over disease is enormously increased; these they term "potencies." Other men term them "dilutions," or "attenuations." The outside scoffer terms them "delusions," but he is positively wrong. By "power" is not meant poison effect which is usually applied to drugs, but *curative* power, for if the potency will cure when the crude drug will not, is it not more powerful? It is the *potency* over disease that must be kept in mind and not poison effect.

Potencies are most commonly made on the centesimal scale. The making of the first potency varies slightly according to the class under which the tincture is prepared, but, as the name of the scale signifies, the strength of the 1st centesimal potency should be the $\frac{1}{100}$ drug power. The subsequent potencies are prepared by taking 1 part of the first potency to 99 parts of alcohol, one part of the 2d to 99 of alcohol and so on, in a well-corked bottle, hold it clinched in the fist and pound on a hair-stuffed base, twelve powerful strokes; this do with each potency.

Thus *Aconite* 3. represents $\frac{1}{1,000,000}$, and *Aconite* 30. 1 followed by 60 ciphers. Yet, as may be seen when figured out, 2,970 drops of alcohol will make this seemingly incredible "high" potency, the potency which Hahnemann claimed gives the best and quickest results. The ignorant are very apt to bring in the element of arithmetical progression here to make the potencies ridiculous, but you see 2,970 drops of alcohol makes the 30th and "the Pacific ocean" or "the universe" is not needed. Also they forget that if arithmetical progression is to be brought in in *quantity* it should also be in *power*. From 4 to 6 tons *energy* have been employed on the 30th potency of 2,970 drops.

Practically, the only difference between the centesimal and the decimal scale is that the latter mounts by tens. Thus, *Aconite* 1x represents 1 part *Aconite* to 9 of the vehicle, *Aconite* 2x, 1-99; *Aconite* 3x, 1-999, and so on, adding one digit for each ascension in the scale; while in the centesimal you add two for each potency—respectively $\frac{1}{10}$ and $\frac{1}{100}$.

The leading remedies have been potentized, by hand, and with alcohol as a vehicle, up to the 200, the 500, and the 1,000th potencies.

Fluxion Potencies.—These are a bone of contention in Homœopathy. They are potencies made with machines—there are different kinds of these machines—with water as a vehicle, and run all the way from the 1,000th to the 1,000,000, or even higher. On the one side it is contended that these potencies represent the insanity of Homœopathy, "faith cure," in other words, and on the other it is contended that they represent such an extreme power that only men of the highest skill in Homœopathy, dare use them, because of the risk of incurring possibly, disastrous results. Be it either way, the beginner in Homœopathy will do well to sail close to the 3d, 6th and 30th potencies; these are curative and also safe.

TRITURATIONS.

Drugs like *Mercurius, Ferrum, Aurum, Stannum,* and many others, are prepared by trituration, but on the decimal scale only. One part of the drug to nine parts of pure recrystallized sugar of milk is triturated in a power-driven mortar for four hours or longer—in first-class pharmacies. This constitutes the, let us say, *Mercurius* 1x trituration. One part of this 1x trit. to nine parts of sugar of milk, triturated for two hours, constitutes the *Mercurius* 2x, or 1-100th, and so on. These triturations run as high as the 60x in a few drugs, but the 1x, 3x and 6x are mostly used. When used in higher potencies these so-called "insolubles" are made into "potencies." This is done by taking one grain of the 6x trituration and dissolving it in 99 minims of distilled water. This is agitated and allowed to stand and again shaken until there is no longer a sediment or anything of the trituration visible. It can then be "run up" as high as desired and prescribed in liquid form, or in medicated pellets, etc. The solution in distilled water is "run up" in pure grain alcohol.

VEHICLES FOR DISPENSING HOMŒOPATHIC MEDICINES.

The most commonly used vehicle for dispensing homœopathic medicine is the cane sugar pellet. Pellets are saturated with the tincture, or dilution, and are then ready for use, and are given on the tongue of the patient; or several dozen pellets may be dissolved in a half-tumblerful of water and a teaspoonful given for a dose.

The dilutions may also be dispensed in the liquid form by putting, say, twenty drops in half a tumblerful of water; teaspoonful a dose.

The triturations, or "powders," are given dry on the tongue in two or three grain doses.

One very popular and convenient form for dispensing homœopathic medicine is in tablets. You can get almost any medicine in this shape and in any reasonable potency, one to three tablets constituting a dose. And in all cases remember that it is not the "strength," or even the frequency of the dose that counts, but its homœopathicity to the case.

TRYING HOMŒOPATHY.

If anyone wants to honestly try Homœopathy let him lay aside prejudice and incredulity, prescribe according to the law of similars, and not imagine that he must give medicine so strong that it can be tasted and smelled. Give the 3d, 6th or 30th potencies and you will have better results with most of the remedies than if you gave the mother tinctures, the 1x or the crude drug.

Some persons argue that the so-called results from the higher potencies of Homœopathy are pure "imagination," but that is not so; in fact, some of our most powerful remedies are practically inert until their latent curative force is developed by prolonged trituration. Of these may be mentioned, among many others, such remedies as *Lycopodium, Carbo vegetabilis* and *Natrum muriaticum*. Give these in the crude form and they are practically inert, but in the 30th potency they exercise a most potent influence over disease when they are indicated.

Hahnemann has been laughed to scorn for claiming for potentized *Natrum mur.* (common table salt) any medicinal power. The skeptical homœopaths of Austria some years ago made a most careful series of experiments, or provings, of this remedy and were reluctantly compelled to admit that potentized salt had a powerful influence on its provers when taken in repeated doses. Such, also, was the experience of von Grauvogl, Director General of the Bavarian army. The case is like that of the "water torture," you can pour a bucket of water over a man and it will not hurt, but let the same come down on him in one spot, a drop at a time, and you have the awful "water torture." So it is with potentized drugs. A child may take a whole vial at once with no harm, but take a dose every hour and you will make a "proving," as the Austrian investigators discovered.

There is one question asked, perhaps, oftener than any other by men trained in other schools of medicine:

"HOW DO YOUR MEDICINES ACT?"

That is a question that has never been answered in an entirely satisfactory manner, and perhaps never will be so answered. The "physiological" action of the various drugs is given in text-books and is well-known to physicians. The physiological action, if carefully noted for its more minute details, is a proving and a guide to the homœopathic use of a drug. So are poison cases.

To illustrate this: A few years ago a child of a prominent homœopathic physician was stricken with what was thought to be malignant scarlet fever, the type that nearly always is fatal. To his surprise the child recovered. He then made an investigation and found that she had chewed the young shoots of the *Ailanthus* tree, she and a little companion, who also developed the same train of symptoms. Later, experiments confirmed this action of the *Ailanthus* on the human body. It was then prepared as a medicine and has *cured* may cases of the type of malignant scarlet fever that before its discovery were nearly always fatal. That was a heroic proving.

Why does *Ailanthus* cause this train of symptoms and why does it cure malignant scarlet fever? Who can answer?

Hahnemann, in *The Organon*, § 28-29, says, "Since this natural law of cure has been verified to the world by every pure experiment and genuine experience, and has thus become an established fact, a scientific explanation of its mode of action is of little importance. I, therefore, place but a slight value upon an attempt at explanation. Nevertheless, the following view holds good as the most probable one, since it is based entirely upon empirical premises."

"We have seen that every disease (not subject to surgery alone) is based upon some particular morbid derangement in the feelings and functions of the vital force, and thus, in the process of a homœopathic cure, by administering a medical potency, chosen exactly in accordance with the similitude of symptoms, a somewhat stronger, similar, artificial, morbid affection is implanted *upon the vital power* deranged by a natural disease; this artificial affection is substituted, as it were, for the weaker similar natural disease (morbid exacerbations), against which the instinctive vital force, now only excited to stronger effort by the drug affection, needs only to direct its increased energy; but owing to its brief duration it will soon be overcome by the vital force, which, liberated first from the natural disease, and finally from the substituted artificial (drug) affection, now again finds itself enabled to continue the life of the organism in health."

So wrote Hahnemann on this subject.

But modern medicine says that disease is of microbic origin. Whether the microbe is the cause or the results of the disease does not alter the universally admitted fact that unless there is a *predisposition* on the part of the patient

HOW DO YOUR MEDICINES ACT? 41

the microbe is powerless. Now it is this predisposition, this morbid derangement in the "vital force" (as Hahnemann puts it), that is the real cause of the disease and it is this that is reached and cured by the potentized remedy. To tell "how" that is done involves an answer to "What is vital force?" "What is life?"

We know we live, but a whole university of scientists cannot tell us how it is done, or what "life" is.

To go deep into this subject one must recognize something more in man than matter; he must recognize mind, spirit or soul. These are the man. Does not the mental state have a most powerful action on the human body? Yet what chemist would seek to "isolate the active principle" of grief or anger, or dread?

And while the mind acts powerfully on the body it is equally true that the states of the body react strongly on the mind. Cognizance is taken of all this in homœopathic practice, and in a careful study of any case, especially of a so-called chronic nature, the mental, as well as the physical symptoms are noted. The potentized drug is, we may say, the soul, or spirit, of the crude drug, and being so, acts on the soul or spirit; on the morbidly deranged "vital force," and so cures the case.

The other theory is that they act as alteratives, diuretics, antipyretics, etc., etc., act physiologically; but when we consider that the physiological action of *Ipecac.* is to cause vomiting, while the small dose will stop vomiting (when not caused by *Ipecac.*), this theory seems untenable.

But, after all is said, the main thing, as Hahnemann intimates, is *to know that these drugs will cure when indicated,* and we must not worry too much over the "how." It is the duty of the physician to heal the sick, and this, when done by drugs, is *always* according to the one healing law. Arsenic acts physiologically the same no matter by whom it is given, or why; so must its curative action be. No one can dispute this self-evident proposition. The homœopath believes that Arsenic (and all drugs) act curatively, if given in very small doses, on diseases which present *similar* symptoms to those which it will cause. That is the whole of Homœopathy in a nutshell. Remember that even before Hippocrates lived that Moses raised up the brazen serpent as a cure for the bitten children of Israel. The older record is something akin to Homœopathy.

PART II.

THERAPEUTICS.

The true homœopathic prescription covers as closely as possible the "totality of the symptoms;" that is to say, the drug whose proving presents the closest resemblance to a given disease is the drug that covers closest the totality of the symptoms.

But during the century in which Homœopathy has been practiced many "keynotes" of the various drugs in their application to the cure of disease have been repeatedly verified and confirmed so that it is now possible to give "guiding symptoms" in many diseases by which the beginner may work very successfully. This section of our book is an effort to give, tersely, the keynotes and guiding symptoms to the various diseases named. To comprehend this take, for example, the first paragraph in the following section: "Abscess or Swellings.—Hot, throbbing, *Belladonna* 3." This means that if you have any abscess or swelling that is *hot,* or throbbing, you give a dose of *Belladonna* 3. Or if it is puffy, and stings—it may be hot also, give *Apis* 3 and so on.

Abscess or "Swellings."—Hot, throbbing, *Belladonna* 3.

Puffy, stinging, *Apis* 3.

Suppurating, pus, *Hepar sulph.* 6.

If slow in healing, constant discharge, watery, *Silicea* 30.

Abscess at the roots of the teeth, *Mercurius viv.* 30.

An occasional dose of *Sulphur* 30th, say, once a week, will prove beneficial in all cases that do not heal rapidly.

See also "Glandular Swellings."

Acne.—*Sulphur* 6. is the best general remedy for acne.

In young persons, *Carbo vegetabilis* 6.

Addison's Disease.—*Arsenicum* 6. may prove beneficial in some cases of this disease. Once a day. This failing, try *Argentum nit.* 6.

Alcoholism.—*Nux vomica* θ, 10 drops, is the classical remedy for the vomiting of alcoholism, twenty drops of *Apocynum cannabinum* decoction in a tumbler of water will put a trembling "old soak" on his feet quicker than any other remedy, according to the late Dr. Stacy Jones. This, however, is not homœopathic, but antidotal, for here is a "removable cause"—too much liquor.

For atony of stomach, *Capsicum* 3.

To allay the craving for alcoholic drinks give

Spiritus glandium quercus (distilled spirit of acorns) 5 drops, twice a day, in half a tumblerful of water.

In delirium tremens, *Hyoscyamus* 3.

Amaurosis.—Appearance of bright spots, *Belladonna* 3.

From abuse of alcohol and tobacco, *Nux vomica* 3.

With no other symptoms, *Tabacum* 30.

Amenorrhœa.—See "Menstruation."

Anæmia.—If patient has been taking iron in any form with no beneficial results stop it and give *Pulsatilla* 3., four times a day, and this especially if the patient feels better in the cool, open air.

Relaxed condition, especially of the female organism, and the patient is always tired and weak, *Aletris* 1.

When patient shivers and wants to be in a warm room, *Arsenicum* 6., three times a day.

Anæmia from loss of vital fluids or the result of lingering illness, *China* 3.

Patient appears full blooded, which is followed by paleness of face, and there is puffiness of the extremities, *Ferrum met.* 6x.

Angina Pectoris.—*Cactus grandiflorus* θ, 1 drop, is the chief homœopathic remedy for this disease.

During intervals it is well to give *Arsenicum* 6. to eradicate the predisposition; a dose every two days.

If caused by straining, or accompanied by rheumatism, *Rhus tox.* 3., twice a day.

If accompanied by blue lips, general coldness and cramps, *Cuprum met.* 6.

Another remarkably effective remedy in this *excruciating* complaint—the italicized word covers the symptom for it—is *Latrodectus mactans*.

An unproved remedy, but one that has given great satisfaction in the treatment of many forms of heart disease, is *Cratægus oxyacantha* θ, in five-drop doses twice a day. It is a fine "heart tonic" and has no bad effects.

Aphthæ (Thrush).—The chief remedy for this disease is *Borax* 6x, twice a day.

If there is a suspicion of syphilitic taint, *Nitric acid* 6.

An occasional dose of *Sulphur* 30., say, once a week, will aid the case if *Borax* does not effect a prompt cure.

Apoplexy.—Very dark red face, stupor, calls for *Opium* 3., every hour until relieved.

Red face, dilated pupils, distended veins, *Belladonna* 3.

Cases that occur without prodroma call for *Laurocerasus* 1x.

In cases of less active congestion and fever, where there have been errors of diet, *Nux vom.* 3.

Appendicitis.—There is a wide difference of opinion on the treatment of this disease, some practitioners claiming 90 per cent. of the cases can be cured with medicine and others that every case is surgical.

Belladonna 3. is called for early in the case when there is severe pain and every jar or touch is painful; give every half hour.

Bryonia 3. is a very useful remedy, called for by soreness and sensitiveness in ileo-cæcal region and disinclination to move. This remedy is probably oftenest indicated.

Arsenicum 6. comes in with sudden sinking of strength, chills and diarrhœa.

Where patient is very restless *Rhus tox.* 3. is indicated.

The free use of olive oil in conjunction with the indicated remedy is also beneficial; indeed some experienced practitioners claim that olive oil alone is all that is needed in the treatment of appendicitis. It is also especially useful if administered as an enema. One English doctor said that in over 500 cases he had never resorted to surgery or lost a case; enemas of oil cured every case.

Arthritis—Gout.—"*Colchicum* is probably the

worst remedy; rely on *Colchicum* and you will get plenty of Bright's disease," says Burnett.

One of the best remedies is *Urtica urens* in five-drop doses of the mother tincture, every two hours, if there is gravel connected with the case, as there generally is.

As an after treatment, if the patient is suffering from the ill effects of alcohol, 10 drops of *Spiritus glandium quercus* (distilled acorns) may be given in water twice a day.

The free use of pure hot water is also useful, especially in the cases of those advanced in years.

Natrum muriaticum 6. is a useful remedy in conjunction with *Urtica urens*.

Another useful remedy is *Ledum;* pains worse from warmth.

Benzoic acid 3. is useful in gouty finger-joints, and Hering says: "The more it is used in gout the more it will be prized."

Asthma.—The most prominent homœopathic remedy for asthma is *Ipecacuanha* 3., *i. e.*, for the spasmodic type with oppression, wheezing and gagging.

Where patient cannot lie down, *Arsenicum* 6. is indicated.

Where caused by gastric disturbances, *Nux vomica* 3.

With yellow, or stringy mucus, *Kali bichromicum* 6.

When there is languor, nausea, vomiting and dyspnœa, *Lobelia inf.* θ.

With great rattling in chest, "moist" asthma, worse in damp weather, *Natrum sulphuricum* 12x. (A good remedy is *Natrum sulph.*)

There is one unproved remedy that has given relief in the worst chronic cases where all else failed and patient was near death, *i. e.*, *Blatta orientalis* 3.

Give remedies every fifteen or thirty minutes, according to the severity of the attack.

An occasional dose of *Sulphur* 30., say, once a week, during intervals will benefit those subject to this disease.

Calcarea carb. 6. where there is a scrofulous taint.

Alternating with rash, *Caladium seg.* 30.

Backache.—The best remedy for simple "backache" is *Pulsatilla* 3.

Where caused by exposure to coldness and dampness, *Rhus tox.* 3.

From dry cold and winds, *Aconite* 3.

Spinal irritation, *Calcarea fluorica* 12x.

Constant aching, no amelioration; in limbs, in sacral region, *Cannabis Indica* 2x.

Lumbago, *Rhus tox.* 3.

Weak back, rickety, scrofulous subjects, *Silicea* 15.

When associated with piles, *Æsculus hippocastanum* 3.

Associated with uterine troubles, *Pulsatilla* 3., or, with brunette, *Sepia* 3.

Another very good back remedy is *Berberis vulgaris*, 3 to 5 drops of the tincture. It has cured many cases of pain in the small of the back or region of the kidneys.

Bilious Attack.—When attack has come on with vomiting of bile, violent headache, and diarrhœa, *Iris versicolor* 3.

With constipation, light stools, sharp pain in liver, frontal headache, *Bryonia* 3.

Pains in the eyes and over them, profuse black tar stool, *Leptandra*.

Aggravated in the morning, morning diarrhœa, *Podophyllum* 3x.

Sharp pains in liver extending to loins, and constipation, *Berberis vulgaris* 6., or θ.

From overindulgence in alcohol or eating, *Nux vomica* 3.

After fat or rich food, *Pulsatilla* 3.

Bladder.—*Cantharis* 3. is the remedy where there is hot urine, pain and constant desire to urinate. Also inability to pass urine.

Evil result following prolonged retention of urine is relieved by *Causticum* 6.

Frequent urging to pass urine, *Apis* 3.

Burning, cutting or sticking pain in urethra,

especially in the female, during and after urinating; frequent desire, *Berberis. vulgaris θ*.

Deposit of red sand, or "brick dust" in urine. *Lycopodium* 6., or, better still, in the 30th potency.

Blood in urine, *Terebinthina* 3.

Bloody from mechanical injuries, *Arnica* 6.

Strangury, *Cantharis* 3.

Urine passed unconsciously, *Argentum nitricum* 6., or, involuntarily, *Causticum* 6.

Scanty urine, *Apis* 6.

Chimaphila umbellata θ in doses of five drops has been highly commended where there is pus in the urine.

Dribbling of urine, *Stramonium* 6.

Inability to retain urine during day, *Ferrum phos.* 6.

Paralysis and inflammation of the bladder, constant desire, only a few drops voided, *Cantharis* 3.

Cases of inability to pass urine, and where catheter has to be used, of years' standing, have been cured by the use of *Solidago virga-aurea* θ in five-drop doses in water, three times a day.

Blood Poisoning.—*Lachesis* 6. is the great remedy for this condition, especially when caused by cuts, as when dissecting or from spoiled meat. Another very useful remedy in depraved blood is *Echinacea* θ in 5 or 10 drop doses.

Boils.—*Hepar sulphuris* 3x is the best general remedy for boils.

Where there is much inflammation and *throbbing*, *Belladonna* 3.

To cure tendency to boils give a daily dose of *Sulphur* 6. for a week or ten days.

Preventive when there is a proneness, *Arnica* 30.

Echinacea θ is also a remedy that has cleared up persistent boil cases when all else failed. It is a great remedy for bad blood, a veritable "blood purifier." Daily, 5 drop doses.

Bones.—Caries of bones, especially if there is a record of syphilis, *Aurum metallicum* 6.

Osseous tumors, *Calcarea fluor.* 12x.

Violent bone pains, *Mercurius viv.* 6.

Periostitis, *Mezereum* 6.

Necrosis, *Silicea* 30.

In all bone disease where there is tuberculosis, or tubercles, an intercurrent dose of *Bacillinum* 30th, 100th or 200th, once a week, will work great good in many cases.

To hasten the uniting of broken bones, *Calcarea phosphorica* 12x.

Another fine remedy for hastening the union of broken or fractured bones is *Symphytum* 3. internally, and the tincture applied externally. The latter application is also very useful for the pain that often persists after the healing process, sometimes for years.

Brain.—*Aconite* 3. is useful in cerebral congestion from cold or exposure.

Bright eyes, flushed face, active delirium, *Belladonna* 3.

Mental torpor, *Helleborus* 3.

Concussion, *Aconite* 3. followed by *Arnica* 3.

Affections from heat of sun, *Glonoinum* 6.

Bronchitis.—*Aconite* 3. is the remedy for early stages and may abort the disease.

Sharp pains in the chest, *Bryonia* 3.

Much rattling of mucus in bronchial tubes, *Ipecac.* 3.

Hoarseness and roughness of throat, loss of voice, *Causticum* 6.

Spasmodic cough, waking the patient up in the night, little expectoration, *Arsenicum album* 6.

Very stringy mucus, *Kali bichromicum* 6.

Threatened suffocation in children who awake with a choking cough, *Tartar emetic* 6x.

Expectoration difficult to raise, *Ammonium carbonicum* 6x.

Chronic bronchitis, *Carbo vegetabilis* 30.

Bruises.—Apply a lotion of 1 part *Arnica* tincture to 20 parts of water; or, rub in *Arnica oil* which is still better, this if the bruise is the result of a severe blow or concussion.

Internally, *Arnica* 3.

Bone bruises, apply *Symphytum* θ, and give same internally in 3d potency.

If the skin is broken apply *Succus Calendulæ*.

Calculus.—Biliary: passage of gall-stones, *Calcarea carb.* 30.; should this fail to relieve within three hours, *Berberis vulg.* θ every 15 minutes. Passage of renal calculi, *Berberis vulg.* θ every 15 minutes.

An old prescription to prevent the formation of gall-stones is a dose of *China* 15. every other day for a month.

Cancer.—The stricter homœopaths all maintain that many cases of cancer can be *cured*, or, at least relieved, by the indicated homœopathic remedy; also that while cutting out the cancer may palliate the trouble for a time, the operation does not remove the cause of the disease, which is constitutional.

In homœopathic literature we find cases of cancer at the root of the tongue cured by *Kali cyanatum* 6.

Indurated glands knotty, *Calc. fluor.* 6.

Arsenicum 6., marked by *burning* pain.

Conium maculatum 3., especially for cancer of the breast, especially when following bruises.

Hydrastis Canadensis 1. has also a reputation in cancer.

Silicea 30. has the reputation of relieving the pain.

Fungus, cauliflower growths, polypoid, *Thuja* 30.

Uranium 6. for cancer of the stomach.
Carbo animalis 6. for hard bluish cancers.
Cholesterine 3x for cancer of the liver.

Guided solely by symptomatology, *Gelsemium, Phosphorus, Phytolacca, Calcarea carb., Lapis albus* (for *hard* tumors) and many other remedies. In no disease must the "totality of the symptoms" be more closely observed and obeyed, if success is to follow the treatment. Many cancers can be cured if the *name* is ignored and the patient's *symptoms* carefully followed.

As an external application the tincture of *Calendula,* or *Succus Calendulæ* (probably the latter is the best) acts favorably in all cases. Also the cerate of *Phytolacca folia,* or *Pine Pitch Ointment;* both of the latter are very useful externally.

All stomach ulcers and cancers are relieved by the free use of pure olive oil internally.

Carbuncle.—The best all-round remedy for typical carbuncle, with black core, is *Tarantula Cubensis* 6.

Other remedies are *Arsenicum* 6., indicated by burning; *Hepar sulphur.* 6., by thickening, and *Lachesis* 6., by symptoms of blood poisoning. Another remedy that has worked wonders in cases of carbuncle is *Echinacea angustifolia* θ in five drop doses, three times a day.

Catalepsy.—*Cannabis Indica* from 1st to 30th potency is the best remedy for this state.

Vertigo, drowsiness, dryness of membranes, *Nux moschata* 30.

If it comes on during monthly periods, *Moschus* 6. is the remedy.

Cataract.—Many cases of this disease have been reported cured by homœopathic medicine; first try *Calcarea fluorica* 12x twice a day for several weeks; if no improvement, then change to *Cannabis Indica* 3. *Fluoric acid* 6. is also useful in this disease.

Catarrh—Colds.—If feverish, restless, anxious, "colds" originating in dry, cold weather, *Aconite* 3.

Thin, watery, excoriating discharge from nose, eyes burning, *Arsenicum* 6.

Pain and pressure, in forehead and at the root of the nose, membranes dry, little or no flowing, *Sticta pul.* 3.

Excoriating discharge, and rawness of throat, *Arum triphyllum* 6.

Nose swollen, red, tears, sweat, better from warmth, thick mucus, *Mercurius* 6.

Flow of clear water from nose, and vesicular eruption, *Natrum muriaticum* 30.

Dull headache, stupid, chilly; also "summer colds," *Gelsemium* 3.

With very much sneezing, and watery eyes, *Allium cepa* 3.

Worse about 3 to 4 in the morning especially in stout persons, *Ammonium carb.* 3.

Stuffed nose, cold on chest, cough painful, *Bryonia* 3.

Always coming on in damp weather, *Dulcamara* 3.

Ozæna, syphilitic catarrh, *Aurum* 6.

Ropy, stringy, mucous discharge, *Kali bichromicum* 6.

Ulceration of nostrils, *Calcarea carb.* 30.

Green fœtid pus, *Mercurius vivus* 6.

Eustachian catarrh, with deafness and tinnitus aurium, *Mercurius dulc.* 3x.

Camphora θ pellets if taken during the preliminary chill will generally abort a cold.

Chest.—Cutting pains, worse by motion and breathing, cough causes pain on chest, *Bryonia* 3.

From dry, cold weather, *Aconite* 3.

Stitches, worse from motion and contact, left side especially affected, *Ranunculus* 3.

Stitch-like pains through the chest, especially when lying down, *Sulphur* 6. Chest seems full of rattling mucus which will not come up, difficulty in breathing, *Tartar emetic* 6.

Chicken-pox.—*Aconite* 3. for the initial stage.

Rhus tox. 3. for eruption.

If case does not progress under the latter remedy change to *Antimonium tartaricum* 6.

Chilblains.—*Pulsatilla* 3. has the reputation of being the best internal remedy for chilblains. *Agaricus mus.* 6. is the remedy when feet itch as if frosted.

Cholera Asiatica.—At the first outset a pellet of the *Rubini Tincture of Camphor* every fifteen minutes for an hour or two will generally abort the disease.

If the attack assumes the form of violent *vomiting,* diarrhœa, thirst, with marked *cold sweat, Veratrum album* 3. is indicated.

Should it take the form of vomiting, purging, rapid prostration with *burning* pains, *Arsenicum* 6x is called for.

Should *cramps* be the most marked symptom the remedy is *Cuprum metallicum* 6.

Should *vomiting* be the most prominent symptom, give *Ipecacuanha* 3.

When case has progressed so far that purging and diarrhœa have ceased and patient lies blue and cold *Carbo vegetabilis* 6. or 30. is the last resort.

As a prophylactic against contracting the disease *Cuprum metallicum* 3x, a dose every other day while exposed, is the thing. It was observed when the disease first invaded Europe that workers in copper never contracted Asiatic cholera, and *Cuprum met.* as a prophylactic has shown its value in many epidemics.

Cholera Infantum.—*Chamomilla* 3. when child wants to be carried, is cross, fretful and stools are a yellowish-green.

Watery diarrhœa, crying, complaining, biting fists, sleepless, *Aconite* 3.

Restlessness, prostration, emaciation, vomiting, thirst, dry skin, are the calls for *Arsenicum* 6.

Attacks brought on by hot weather, or in attacks where child lies still, *Bryonia* 3.

Marked cold sweat, *Veratrum album* 3.

Rumbling in bowels, no thirst, *Pulsatilla* 3.

Blue rings about the eyes, vomiting, green, *Ipecacuanha* 3.

Unconscious, yet with staring eyes, milk vomited in curds, spasms, *Æthusa* 3.

Stupor, broken by screams, *Apis* 3.

Fat, flabby, fair children, with large heads, which sweat unnaturally, will be benefitted by *Calcarea carbonica* 30.

If soreness be prominent, *Rheum* 3.

Cramps, *Cuprum* 6.

During teething, *Calcarea phos.* 6x.

Caused by exposure to dry cold, begin with *Aconite* 3.

Stools slimy, bloody, *Mercurius vivus* 6.

Bloody flux, *Mercurius corrosivus* 6.

If any case lingers too long give an occasional dose of *Sulphur* 30.

Cholera Morbus.—If caused by ice cream, ice water or green fruit; burning, thirst, *Arsenicum* 6.

If nausea and vomiting predominate, *Ipecacuanha* 3.

Severe diarrhœa, cramps, cold sweat, *Veratrum album* 3.

Milk-white tongue, overloaded stomach. *Antimonium crudum* 6.

See also "Diarrhœa."

Chorea.—*Agaricus muscarius* 1x is one of the most prominent remedies in chorea; twitching and jerking are its keynotes. Some physicians claim that *Agaricus* 2x is preferable.

Jerking about the arms, *Hyoscyamus* 3.

From mental cause, *Ignatia* 3.

From worms, *Cina* 3.

With cold, damp feet, *Calcarea carbonica* 6.

Movements very rapid, stammering, *Stramonium* 6.

During teething, *Calcarea phosphorica* 6x.

Colds.—See Catarrh.

Colic.—*Colocynthis* 3. covers most cases; pain makes patient bend double; if this does not give him quick relief try *Dioscorea villosa* 1.

Another remedy is *Magnesia phosphorica* 6x in hot water; this is especially for neuralgic-like pain.

Navel violently retracted, great pain, **Plumbum** 6.

In teething children and children generally, *Chamomilla* 3.

Flatulent colic, *Chamomilla* 3.

Flatulent colic in spare, dark subjects with constipation, *Nux vom.* 3.

From indigestion, *Nux vomica* 3.

Lead colic, *Opium* 6.

Constipation.—Large, dry stools; patient irritable and rheumatic, *Bryonia* 3.

For days no desire for stool; constipation very obstinate, *Alumen* 30.

Urgent desire, but with effort the desire passes away, *Anacardium* 3.

Frequent ineffectual urging, sedentary life; also in cases of those who have taken much medicine, purgatives, etc., *Nux vomica* 3.

Sulphur 6x and *Nux vomica* 3. in alternation, say, every two hours, has cured many cases of the ill with no very marked indications.

Where there seems to be actual paralysis of the bowels, *Opium* 30. is the remedy.

Long, very slender stools, *Phosphorus* 30.

With colic, *Plumbum* 6.

Associated with violent, dry coughs, *Nitric acid* 6.

Associated with piles, *Collinsonia* 3.

With rumbling in the bowels, and belching of wind, *Lycopodium* 30.

Difficult expulsion of even a soft stool, *Platina* 30.

Where stool actually crumbles, *Natrum mur.* 30.

Kneading the stomach, drinking freely of pure water, and the use of olive oil is beneficial in habitual constipation in addition to the indicated remedy. Also going to stool at a regular hour daily.

The regular use of cathartics is one of the best means of *inducing* constipation. A dry "pill" or purgative has no moisture, so to force a stool it must draw moisture from the body; keep this up long enough and the constipation is worse and possibly appendicitis not far off.

Consumption.—Tuberculosis if taken in time can very often be cured by homœopathic medicines. The chief remedy, according to the late Dr. J. Compton Burnett (see his work, *New Cure for Consumption*), is *Bacillinum,* never to be given lower than the 30th and preferably in the 100th potency and *not oftener than once a week;* it is to be given with the other remedies as indicated. Even in advanced cases this remedy will give patient relief and greater ease.

Phosphorus 3. or 30. is indicated by blood streaked sputum, hectic fever, hoarseness and evening aggravation; but *do not give it too often,* once a day at most.

Calcarea carb. 6. to 30. is indicated in lumpy,

yellow-green, purulent matter; sensitive to cold; perspires; easily fatigued.

Sulphur 6. to 30. is especially indicated when the skin is unhealthy, dry and scaly.

Constant sense of fermentation in stomach, *Lycopodium* 30.

Hæmorrhages of bright red blood, *Nitric acid* 6. or *Ipecac.* 3.

In suppurative stage, profuse night sweats, *Silicea* 6. or 30.

Where *weakness* is very prominent, *Stannum metallicum* 6.; suitable also where catarrhal states have preceded.

Arsenicum iodide 12x is indicated where there is a tendency to diarrhœa and marked hectic fever.

If blood is dark *Hamamelis* 1x, is indicated.

Tuberculosis in any part of the body will be benefitted by infrequent doses of the *Bacillinum* 30. in connection with the remedy indicated.

Always remember that a careful summary of all the symptoms, in this, as in all other diseases, is the true guide to the curative medicine; ignore name of disease.

There seems to be a returning to the old belief that this is a hereditary or constitutional disease, if so, it should be met by skilled homœopathic treatment in childhood.

Convulsions.—Face blue, clenched fingers, cold sweat, *Cuprum met.* 6.

Face flushed, *Belladonna* 3.
Face pale, *Zincum met.* 6.
From mental causes, *Ignatia* 3.
Nightmare, *Pæonia officinalis* 3.
When one convulsion follows another with alarming frequency give *Cicuta virosa* 3.
In emergency turn patient at once on *left* side.

Cough.—Short, dry, irritating cough; cough during sleep, *Aconite* 3.
Chronic, with profuse expectoration of phlegm, *Allium sativum* 3.
Child awakes gasping and coughing with chest full of phlegm, rattling, difficult breathing, *Antimonium tartaricum* 6. (*Tartar emetic.*)
Dry, painful cough, patient holds hands to chest, *Bryonia* 3.
Teasing, tickling, dry cough, which ceases when patient goes to bed, better from warm air, *Rumex crispus* 3.
Cough which causes involuntary spurting of urine, *Causticum* 6.
Violent cough with *clear*, ropy mucus, *Coccus cacti* 6.
Violent cough with stringy, ropy, *yellow* mucus, *Kali bichromicum* 6.
Hard, barking cough, like a saw driven through board, croup, *Spongia* 3.
Whooping cough, ending in vomiting, *Drosera rotundifolia* 3.

Cough ending with choking and gagging, *Hepar sulphuris* 6.

Dry cough while lying down, but relieved by arising, *Hyoscyamus* 3.

Raw, scraping cough, nose sore, throat raw, sweat, *Mercurius vivus* 6.

Violent cough jarring the head, little or no expectoration, *Nux vomica* 3.

Loose cough, with much mucus (in blondes), *Pulsatilla* 30.

Spasmodic cough, coming on in the night, waking the patient from sleep, ending in bringing away a little phlegm, *Arsenicum alb.* 6x.

Dry cough, excited by smoke, cold air, talking or reading, *Mentha piperita* 30.

Violent dry cough, with constipation, *Nitric acid* 3.

Cough, especially excited by dry, cold air, *Aconite* 3.

Cough excited by lying down, *Conium maculatum* 3.

Nervous, hysterical coughs, *Corallium rubrum* 30.

Incessant, tickling cough, *Sanguinaria nitrate* 3x.

Nervous cough, where the more the patient coughs the greater is the incitation to cough, *Ignatia* 30.

Cough ending in gagging and vomiting, *Ipecac.* 3.

With marked, yellow color of expectoration, *Kali sulphuricum* 12x.

Markedly spasmodic, associated with severe pain, *Magnesia phosphorica* 12x in hot water.

With clear, watery, or white and frothy expectoration, *Natrum muriaticum* 30.

Associated with sour acid conditions, *Natrum phosphoricum* 12x.

Associated with bilious or jaundiced conditions, *Natrum sulphuricum* 12x.

Cramps.—In general, *Cuprum metallicum* 6. is the best remedy or *Magnesia phos.* 6x.

With cold sweat, diarrhœa and vomiting, *Veratrum album* 3.

Writer's cramp, *Gelsemium* 3.

Croup.—For the fever, hot, dry skin and restlessness, *Aconite* 3. This remedy is indicated in the beginning of every case of croup.

A hard, barking cough, and breathing sounding harsh, almost like a saw driven through a board, indicates *Spongia* 3.

Where the cough is loose, *Hepar sulphur.* 6. is indicated.

Many successful practitioners have given these three remedies in the order named above in rotation, a dose every hour, with wonderful success. Where the chest seems full of phlegm, child chokes and gasps, *Tartar emetic* 6.

Aconite 3., *Hepar sulph.* 6. and *Spongia* 3. following each other every 15 minutes has saved many a case of uncomplicated croup. This trio is almost specific.

Debility.—Men break down, brain fag, nervous, cry like children, *Kali phosphoricum* 6x.

Debility from loss of blood, or from long illness, *China* 3.

Sexual debility, Phosphoric acid 3.

Patient so weak that he gradually slips down towards foot of bed, *Muriatic acid* 6.

Debility associated with grief, *Ignatia* 3.

Dentition.—Emaciated, thin children with open fontanelles; slow in teething, *Calcarea phosphorica* 6x.

Vomiting large curds of milk, *Æthusa* 3.

Spongy gums, teeth decay very early, *Kreosotum* 3.

For the general irritability of teething, normal children, *Chamomilla* 3. is the sovereign remedy.

Feverishly bright eyes, high fever, brain involved, convulsions, *Belladonna* 3.

Fever, hot, dry skin, and great restlessness, *Aconite* 3.

Diabetes.—Profuse quantities of pale, colorless urine, *Phosphoric acid* 3.

Sugar in urine a very marked feature, *Uranium* 3x.

Rhus aromatica θ ten drops to a teaspoonful of water is claimed will cure diabetes.

Lactic acid 3. is an excellent remedy.

Tube casts, uric acid, *Plumbum iodide* 6x.

Diarrhœa.—For simple uncomplicated cases of diarrhœa, *Chininum arsenicosum* 6x will suffice.

Summer diarrhœa; frequently watery stools with griping pains, *China* 1. or 3.

Stools small, dark colored, very offensive, patient restless, suffers anguish, great thirst, *Arsenicum* 6.

Genuine "bellyache," cold sweat, *Veratrum album* 3.

The stool and patient seem sour, *Rheum* 3.

Straining, pain, never-get-done feeling, *Mercurius vivus* 6.

Stools bloody, "bloody flux," *Mercurius corrosivus* 6.

Very watery, yellow, gushing, *Croton tiglium* 6.

Pain bends patient double, *Colocynthis* 3.

In children, scrofulous, who sweat much about the head, *Calcarea carbonica* 30.

Uneasy weakness about rectum, fæces passes with flatus, *Aloe* 3.

Morning diarrhœa, brown watery, urgent, waking patient from sleep, *Rumex* 3.

Aggravation in morning and tendency to anal prolapsus. Especially in bilious temperament, *Podophyllum* 3. See also "Cholera Morbus."

Diphtheria.—Pain on swallowing and white deposit in throat, *Kali muriaticum* 6x.

When disease first appears on left side of throat, great fetor, gangrenous tendency, *Lachesis* 6.

Septic condition, face dark, typhoid state, *Baptisia* 1.

Mercurius cyanatus 6., when tongue is of dark brown color, or blackish.

Marked weakness, blood dark, nose-bleed, *Muriatic acid* 6.

Aching all over, throat very sore, *Phytolacca* 3.

Echinacea angustifolia θ ten drops, in water, is a favorite diphtheria remedy with many practitioners, especially for marked septic conditions.

Much œdema, throat glossy red, suppression of urine, *Apis mel.* 3.

Very tough exudation, yellow tongue, *Kali bichromicum* 6x.

Pineapple juice is an excellent adjuvant in every case. The juice tends to clear the membrane.

Dropsy.—One of the best general remedies for dropsy is twenty drop doses twice a day of the *Decoction of Apocynum cannabinum.*

Dropsy following scarlet fever, swollen puffy feet, *Apis mellifica* 3.

With hæmorrhage from kidneys, *Terebinthina* 3.

Oozing serum, waxy skin, thirst, ulceration, *Arsenicum* 6.

When legs are much swollen, much thirst, *Acetic acid* 1.

Dysentery.—The chief remedy for this complaint, if it be bloody in character, is *Mercurius corrosivus* 6.

Burning, thirst, and severe prostration, *Arsenicum* 6.

Tympanitic distension, *Lycopodium* 30.

Chronic, *Sulphur* 30.

If fever be present an intercurrent dose of *Aconite* 3.

Nausea, vomiting, passages of blood, *Ipecacuanha* 3.

Dysmenorrhœa.—Dark colored, fitful flow, delayed, *Pulsatilla* 3.

Clotted blood, severe headache, nausea, uterine cramps, *Cocculus* 3.

Neuralgic-like pains, relief from warmth, *Magnesia phosphorica* 12x.

Headache precedes, sharp labor-like pains, *Cimicifuga* 3.

Spasmodic cases, bearing down pains, hysterical, *Caulophyllum* 1.

Congestive, *Belladonna* 3.
Dark rings about the eyes, worse in the morning, bilious, yellow, *Sepia* 3.
See also "Menstruation."
Dyspepsia.—Flatulent, acrid, heartburn, loose bowels, *Carbo vegetabilis* 30.
From indigestible food, tongue brown at the back, cramping or spasmodic pain, flatulence, vomiting, constipation, *Nux vomica* 3.
Feeling as of stone in the stomach, *Bryonia* 3.
Feeling as if the stomach were loaded with undigested, hard boiled eggs, *Abies nigra* 3.
In whiskey drinkers, *Nux vomica* 3. or *Capsicum* 3.
In beer drinkers, *Kali bichromicum* 6x.
From starchy foods, *Natrum muriaticum* 30.
From eating rich or fat food, heartburn, *Pulsatilla* 3.
Tongue milky white, *Antimonium crudum* 6.
Acid risings, dyspepsia in the aged, *Kali carbonicum* 6.
Hungry, but a few mouthfuls satiate, fulness, gas, *Lycopodium* 30.
Burning in the stomach, *Arsenicum* 6.
Pain comes on some time *after* eating though immediately after eating there is relief, *Anacardium* 3.
Pine apple juice is an excellent all-round remedy.

Yellow, slimy tongue, sodden face, "goneness," *Hydrastis Canadensis* 3.

Chronic cases, sour risings, with canine hunger, *Phosphorus* 30.

Ear.—Discharges of blood and matter from the ear, *Capsicum* 6.

Red, burning, itching ears, *Agaricus muscarius* 6.

Inflammation of middle ear, after exposure to dry cold, at the beginning pain, restlessness, anxiety, *Aconite* 3.

Catarrhal inflammation of the middle ear, *Kali muriaticum* 6x.

Puffy, swollen ears, *Apium virus* 6.

Earache, *Pulsatilla* 3., or else a pledget of cotton saturated with *Mullein oil* stuffed in the ears; or *Plantago* θ may be applied locally.

Acute otitis, *Belladonna* 3. or, if brought on by dry cold or sudden change in the weather, *Aconite* 3.

Otitis externa, *Pulsatilla* 3.

Yellowish-green discharge, *Pulsatilla* 3.

Infantile earache, *Chamomilla* 3.

Thin, acrid discharges, *Mercurius vivus* 6.

Suppuration, *Silicea* 30.

Deafness in Eustachian tubes, cracking in the ears, *Kali muriaticum* 6x.

Eczema, *Rhus toxicodendron* 3.; this failing, *Mezereum* 30.

Polypus in the scrofulous, *Calcarea carbonica* 30. In all others, *Thuja* 30.
Boils, *Hepar sulphuris* 6.
Bran-like scales, *Arsenicum* 6.
Moist, sticky eruptions, *Graphites* 6.
Roaring noises, *China* 3.
Cracking in ears. Hold nose tight with thumb and fingers, close mouth and then blow breath; this process will open the tubes. Also, *Kali muriaticum* 6x.

For deafness, unless from some incurable cause, like perforation, drop four or five minims of *Mullein oil* in the ear.

For deafness caused by blocking of the Eustachian tube, *Mercurius* 6. If it does not yield after a week of this, *Hydrastis* 1.

Ecchymosis—"Black and Blue."—Whenever there is a blow from which "black and blue" spots follow, take *Arnica* 30, *internally*.

Eczema.—On face or genital organs, *Croton tiglium* 6.

Moist in bends of joints, between fingers, palms of hands, behind ears, etc., *Graphites* 6.

Itching and burning, *Arsenicum* 6.; if scaly skin, *Sulphur* 30.; if red, *Rhus tox.* 3.

Dry, irritative eczema, *Alumina* 6.
Eczema of backs of hands, *Bovista* 6.
Eczema of chin in males, *Cicuta vir.* 3.
Yellow, crusty, *Sulphur* 30.

On scrotum, *Hepar sulphuris* 6.

Eczema capitis, *Kali muriaticum* 12x; also *Oleander* 6.

Chalk-like crusts, *Calcarea carbonica* 30.

An unproved remedy, "*Skookum chuck*" 3x (the salts of Medical lake), has been prescribed most successfully in many bad cases of eczema, palmaritis, psoriasis, etc., etc. It is really a great remedy for such skin ills.

Some practitioners claim that *Rhus tox.* 30. is the *best* remedy for all forms of this disease.

Emissions, Seminal.—Milky urine, system relaxed, debility, no erection, *Phosphoric acid* 3.

Very frequent emissions with violent erections, *Picric acid* 6.

Loss of memory, nervous prostration, *Anacardium orientale* 6.

Complete breakdown, mentally and physically, *Kali phosphoricum* 6x.

Epilepsy.—Probably the best general remedy for recent epilepsy is *Œnanthe crocata* 3., violent convulsions, foaming at the mouth.

Another excellent remedy is *Cicuta virosa* 6., frightful contortions; also in infants.

When attacks come with great frequency, *Artemesia vulgaris* 1x.

With frightful cramps and spasms, face blue, *Cuprum met.* 6.

When brought on by mental causes *only*, *Ignatia* 30.

Chronic epilepsy in general, *Rana bufo* 6.

When chronic, spasms, followed by prolonged sleep, *Opium* 6.

Brought on by masturbation, *Rana bufo* 6.

In scrofulous subjects, *Calcarea carbonica* 30.

Erysipelas.—Shining, dark red skin, *Belladonna* 3.

The vesicular variety, *Rhus tox.* 3.

In simple acute cases, *China θ*.

Puffy swelling, stinging pains, *Apium virus* 6.

Frequently recurring, especially about the face, *Graphites* 6.

Fever, thirst, prostration, burning, *Arsenicum* 6.

Going on to gangrene, *Crotalus horridus* 6.

Eyes.—Dry, inflamed, intolerance of light, *Belladonna* 3.

Inflammation brought on by exposure to dry cold, *Aconite* 3.

Swelling, with acrid discharge, *Rhus tox.* 3.

Inflamed lids, profuse excoriating discharge, *Euphrasia* 3.

Conjunctivitis, "pus eye," eyelids glued together in the morning, *Mercurius* 6.; this failing, *Argentum nitricum* 6.

Corneal ulceration, *Kali muriaticum* 6x.

Gonorrhœal ophthalmia, *Kali sulphuricum* 6x.

Styes, *Pulsatilla* 3.

Cataract, or opacity of cornea, *Calcarea fluorica* 6x; this failing, *Cannabis sativa* 1x.

Aching eyes from eye strain, *Actea racemosa* 3.; or *Ruta graveolens* 6. for dim vision from overuse of eyes.

Eye trouble from syphilis, *Aurum metallicum* 6.

Severe shooting pains back of eyes, *Cedron* 6.

Great puffiness under the eyes, *Apis mellifica* 3, or *over* the eyes, *Kali carb.* 30.

Eyes unnaturally dry, *Alumina* 30.

Angles of eyelids sore and raw, *Graphites* 6.

Strumous ophthalmia, *Sulphur* 30.

Twitching of eyelids, *Agaricus muscarius* 6.

Rheumatic pains in the eyes, *Bryonia* 3.

Inflammation following presence of foreign bodies, or hurts, also from cold, *Aconite* 3.

Lachrymal fistula, *Silicea* 30.

"Watery" eyes, *Euphrasia* 3.

Feet.—Callosities on the soles, *Antimonium crudum* 6.

Waxy and swollen, *Apis mellifica* 3.

Nocturnal itching, *Ledum* 3.

Offensive foot sweat, *Silicea* 30.

Soles of feet burn, *Sulphur* 30.

Pain in heels, *Cyclamen* 30.

Cold, damp, clammy feet, *Calcarea carb.* 30.

Pain in great toe, *Dulcamara* 3.

Oozing soreness between the toes, *Graphites* 6.

Chilblains, *Pulsatilla* 3., or *Agaricus* 6.

Rheumatism beginning in feet and traveling upwards, *Ledum* 3.

Cramp, *Cuprum met.* 6.

Swollen, tender, with foul sweat, *Petroleum* 3. or *Silicea* 30.

Feel sprained, *Rhus tox.* 3.

"Fidgety" feet, *Zincum* 6.

Ankles give way, *Chamomilla* 3.

Gangrene.—*Echinacea angustifolia* θ is the best remedy to arrest this condition, give it in ten drop doses internally.

Senile gangrene; skin shrivelled, worse from external heat, *Secale* 3.

Another remedy that has proved successful is *Lachesis* 6., in traumatic gangrene; also *Crotalus* 6. with swelling, foul odor, with black or bluish discoloration.

Gastralgia.—Cramp-like, spasmodic pain, *Nux vom.* 3. every two hours.

Burning pain, *Arsenicum alb.* 3. every two hours.

Pain with catarrhal inflammation of the alimentary canal. Frequent eructations, *Bismuthum* 1x every hour.

Spasmodic pains compelling patient to bend double, *Colocynth.*

Cramps with sour stomach, *Carbo veg.*

Glandular Swelling.—At the commencement, *Belladonna* 3.

If in submaxillary gland, *Arum tri.* 6.
If suppuration threatens, *Mercurius sol.* 6.
If suppuration has actually taken place, *Hepar sul. cal.* 6.
Glandular indurations, *Clematis* 3.
Pains extending to the abdomen, *Iodum* 30.

Goitre.—It has been asserted and confirmed in a large number of cases that *Fucus vesiculosis* θ in half teaspoonful doses, three times a day, will cure many cases of goitre in those under thirty years of age. Treatment must be persisted in for several months.

The other remedies are *Acid fluoricum* 6. and *Calcarea carbonica* 30. in scrofulous subjects. In old hard goitres, *Spongia* 3., four times a day, for weeks.

When there is irritability of the nervous system, emaciation but with good appetite, *Iodum* 30.

Gonorrhœa.—Yellow or greenish discharge, *Natrum sulphuricum* 12x.

For sexual excitement, *Cantharis* 3.
Chordee, *Cannabis Indica* 1x.
Fever, *Aconite* 3.
Much inflammation, *Mercurius vivus* 6.

Thick yellow discharge, profuse, scalding, erections; when the prostate gland is affected, *Thuja* 3.

Fig warts, condylomata, sycotic dyscrasia, *Thuja* 30.

Profuse discharge, little pain, *Pulsatilla* 3.
Chronic cases, *Natrum mur.* 30.
In women, after acute stage, *Sepia* 3.
In all cases an occasional dose of *Sulphur* 30., with selected remedy, will prevent disease from becoming violent.
Strict homœopathic treatment admits of no injections.
To re-establish discharge after suppression by external means, which is *no cure, Sulphur* 30.
Testicles swell in consequence of suppression of discharge, *Pulsatilla* 3.

Gout.—Burnett claims that *Urtica urens* θ, five drops in a wineglassful of hot water, every three hours, will give quick relief, as it expels the gravel, uric acid, etc. The same author claims that *Spiritus glandium quercus* θ, ten drops in water, for ten days, will antidote the ill effects of alcohol and allay craving for liquor.

Where patient is chilly and cannot stand the seashore, *Natrum mur.* 12x.

Where heart is weak, *Aurum muriaticum* 3x.

Lycopodium 30. is indicated by red sand in urine.

The free use of hot water in the aged and spare is beneficial. Juicy fruit is also beneficial in all cases.

As for *Colchicum*, Burnett says: "Rely on

Colchicum in gout and you will get plenty of Bright's disease." This, however, refers to routine treatment. *Colchicum* 3. is indicated where there are gastric or cardiac complications.

Arnica 3. is indicated when patient is abnormally fearful when any one approaches his foot.

Hæmorrhage.—From bowels, dark blood, *Hamamelis* 3x.

Bright colored blood, *Ipecac.* 3x.

Black and stringy (Metrorrhagia), *Crocus sat.* θ.

Increased by least motion and of a bright red color, *Erigeron* θ.

Hæmorrhoids.—Bleeding piles, *Hamamelis* 3.

Blind piles, in spare, constipated persons who lead sedentary lives, *Nux vomica* 3. morning, and *Sulphur* 30. evening.

Feeling as of sharp sticks in the rectum (from bleeding), pain in the back, and prolapse, *Æsculus hippocastanum* 3.

Inertia of bowels, constipation, *Collinsonia Canadensis* 1.

With anal fissure, stools large and knotty, *Graphites* 6.

With mucus, like white of eggs, which oozes out, *Antimonium crudum* 6.

With intense itching, *Ratanhia* 3.

The cure is greatly aided by the use of suppositories in conditions indicated above, of

Hamamelis, Æsculus hip., Collinsonia, Ratanhia or combinations of same. (See various homœopathic price currents.)

Hands and Fingers.—Hands chapped from exposure or working in water, wash clean with warm water and soap before retiring and then thoroughly rub with *Calendula ointment*.

Hands with deep, hard, oozing cracks, *Graphites* 6.

Excoriating between fingers, *Graphites* 6.

Itching, burning, trembling, *Agaricus musc.* 3.

Cold, clammy hands, *Fluoric acid* 6.

Hands dry and rough, *Natrum carb.* 6.

Swollen finger-joints, gouty, *Benzoic acid* 6x; otherwise, *Ledum palustre* 3.

Tips of fingers cracked and rough, *Petroleum* 3.

Fingers feel dead, *Calcarea carb.* 30.

"Wrist drop," *Plumbum* 30.

Hay Fever.—The nearest approach to the typical hay fever is to be found in the proving of *Arundo mauritanica* 3x, and it has proved to be very satisfactory in practice.

Where with lachrymation there is swelling and excoriation, *Naphthalin* 3x.

Much sneezing, but little discharge, *Sabadilla* 3.

When disease is complicated with asthma, *Ipecac.* 3.

Arsenicum 6. is indicated when with the usual hay fever symptoms a *burning* sensation is marked.

Headache.—*Throbbing and fulness*, light is painful, least jar is painful, *Belladonna* 3.

Congestive headache, very violent, bursting, *Melilotus alba* 1x.

Hot, red face, frontal headache, worse from motion, *Bryonia* 3.

Chronic headache in back of head, *Nitric acid* 6.

Pain over one eye, *Sepia* 3.

Chronic headache, with melancholia, *Zincum* 30.

Neuralgic headache, very painful, *Spigelia* 3.

Chronic headache, better from warmth, *Silicea* 30.

Sick headache, that increases and decreases with the rising and setting of the sun, *Sanguinaria Canadensis* 3.

Blurring, blinding, sour vomit, *Iris versicolor* 3.

Sick headache, in women, brought on by shopping or any departure from usual routine, *Epiphegus Virginiana* 3.

Chronic, dull, associated with constipation, *Plumbum* 6.

Headache from alcohol, *Nux vomica* 3., *Bryonia* 3., or *Acetic acid* 3.

Headache in one spot, *Ignatia* 3.
Dull, passive, stupid headache, *Gelsemium* 3.
Headache from sun heat, *Glonoinum* 3.
Relieved by bandaging, or deep in the brain, vertigo, *Argentum nitricum* 6.
As from heavy weight on top of the head, *Phellandrium aquaticum* 3x.
One-sided headache, *Calcarea carb.* 6.
Excruciating pain, shifting and intermittent, *Magnesia phos.* 12x.
"Bilious" headache, *Chionanthus Virginica* 1x.
Headache of compositors, bookkeepers, reporters, clerks, etc., of those who have to work much under gas light, *Glonoinum* 6.

Heart.—Hughes says of *Digitalis* that its poison effect is to cause a "dead heart in a living body." It is homœopathically indicated in palpitation, slow, irregular or intermittent heart beats; fears sometimes heart will stop beating, cardiac dropsy. Gloomy sadness is a characteristic of the *Digitalis* patient.

Palpitation and pain, as though the heart were bound in iron; carditis; *Cactus grandiflorus* 1x or θ.

Beat strong, irregular, pain radiates from the heart, breathing painful; burning pain, *Arsenicum* 6.

Carditis, pericarditis, rheumatic heart, sharp

pains from heart into arm or down spine; tumultuous heart beats, *Spigelia* 3.

In heart affections where there are stitching pains, and numb or tingling fingers, *Aconite* 3.

Heart troubles following rheumatism are well met by *Kalmia latifolia* 3.

Heart affections brought on by overexertion, as in athletics, *Arnica* 3.

Suffocative feeling when lying flat on the back, *Spongia* 3.

Tobacco heart, *Kalmia latifolia* 3.

Heart beat frequent, spasmodic; painless twitching of cardiac muscles, *Argentum metallicum* 6x.

One of the best general heart remedies is *Cratægus oxyacantha* θ, in five-drop doses, two or three times a day. If the term be permissible it seems to be an excellent "heart tonic," useful in nearly all cases.

Hernia.—While this disease is usually treated solely by mechanical or surgical methods, nevertheless *Nux vomica* 3. will prove to be of very great benefit to the patient in all cases and will cure many of them.

Hiccough.—*Ginseng* θ will cure nearly every case; if it fails try *Nux vomica* 3.

Hoarseness.—See **Voice.**

Hydrocephalus.—It is always well to begin treatment of this disease with a dose of *Bacilli-*

num 30th or 100th, preferably the latter, and to continue it during treatment, one dose a week, this in connection with the indicated remedy.

In acute cases *Belladonna* 3. where there are flushed face, wild eyes and grinding of teeth.

Where child lies stupid, with no marked symptoms, *Helleborus* 3.

Rolls head from side to side, or bores it into the pillow; screams occasionally; jerking muscles; fidgety feet, *Zincum* 6.

Urine scanty, child bores its head in the pillow and occasionally utters piercing screams, *Apis mel.* 3.

Calcarea phosphorica 6x, is indicated in cases attended by retarded dentition.

Hydrophobia.—Let any one who has been bitten by a supposedly rabid animal take *Arsenicum* 6., twice a day, for a week.

Hysteria.—*Ignatia* 3. is one of the chief remedies in this puzzling complaint. Patient alternately laughs and cries.

When fainting fits are a concomitant, *Moschus* 3. is the remedy.

Associated with nymphomania, *Platina* 6.

Associated with excessive irritability, *Valeriana* 6x.

Globus hystericus, *Nux moschata* 30.

Sensation of a ball coming up into the throat; worse from nervous excitement, *Asafœtida* 3x.

Influenza—Grippe.—The remedy for this epidemic—when it is epidemic—seems to change from time to time. The following medicines will best meet the varying symptoms:

Aconite 3.—When patient is very restless, anxious, with *fear*. Generally the best remedy to start with.

Gelsemium 3. where there is marked languor, loss of muscular power, shivering and weariness. Patient dull and sluggish.

Eupatorium perf. 3.—The great indication for this remedy is bone-breaking character of the pain.

Bryonia 3.—This patient wants to lie absolutely quiet for he is worse from slightest motion.

Arsenicum alb. 6.—Is called for in all cases characterized by the sudden onset of the disease and the rapid prostration that follows. Its symptoms are intense, hot, burning, restless, etc.

Mercurius 6.—Is called for where there is shivering and hot spells, "goose-flesh," sour, oily, sweaty condition, slimy mouth, nose red and swollen, eyes red. Better from warmth, cough.

Sabadilla 3.—The peculiarities of this drug are the creeping *upwards* of sensations; drowsy in day time and chilly toward evening, joints painful. Skin dry and cough appears on lying down. Much sneezing and lachrymation.

Natrum sulph. 12x is said by many to be the "grippe specific," especially where the disease was contracted in *damp,* cold weather. Get the tablets, 3 a dose, four times a day.

Intermittent Fever.—Absence of thirst during chill and fever, rush of blood to the head, thirst with sweat and debility, *China* 3.

Chill and fever not distinctly developed, commingle with each other, heat, burning, great thirst, *Arsenicum alb.* 6.

Great thirst before and during chill, but none in fever, or following it; headache, profuse sweat, *Natrum mur.* This remedy is also very suitable in lingering cases.

Oppressed breathing, nausea, vomiting, fever long lasting, *Ipecac.* 3. Especially useful in epidemics.

Where backache and bone pains are prominent, "break bone fever," *Eupatorium perfoliatum* 3.

In young weakly persons who flush easily; during the heat, distension of blood-vessels and headache; chill apt to come on about three or four in the morning, *Ferrum met.* 3x.

Pale face, long-lasting chill, cold sweat on forehead, extremities cold, exhaustion, *Veratrum album* 3.

Where sweat comes with the fever, *Capsicum* 3.

Occurring in persons returning from warm climates, obscure cases; marked regularity of appearance of symptoms, *Cedron* 3.

Where there is marked gastric and bilious disturbance, *Nux vomica* 3.

Where spleen is involved, *Ceanothus Americana* θ, in five-drop doses. Wherever the spleen in involved *Ceanothus Amer.* will be found to be an "organ remedy" according to the late Dr. J. C. Burnett.

In cases where much quinine has been taken and the patient is something of a "wreck" *Natrum mur.* 30. will often work wonders.

The best time to give the medicine in this disease is during the remission.

Irritation—Pruritus.—Itching worse in heat at night followed by dry burning, *Sulphur* 30.

Itching of the vulva, *Caladium seg.* 3. every two hours.

Itching burning rash alternating with asthma, *Calad. seg.* 30.

Flea bite like eruption with intolerable itching, *Agaricus mus.* 3.

Intense and recurring itching in same spot, *Mezereum* 3.

Jaundice.—Skin dirty, offensive sweat, region of liver sore, *Mercurius vivus* 6.

Marked pain under right shoulder blade, *Chelidonium majus* θ, in five-drop doses. An "organ remedy" for the liver.

Great thirst, worse from motion, *Bryonia* 3.
Very malignant, *Phosphorus* 3.
Aching and soreness of liver with profuse black, tarry stool, *Leptandra* θ.
Clay-like stools, urine dark, bitter, bilious headache. *Chionanthus Vir.* θ, two drop doses.

Kidneys.—"Infamous odor of urine when first passed, which is increased by standing," *Cina* 3.
Nephritis, inflammation of the kidneys, bloody urine, *Terebinthina* 3.
Puffy swelling, dull pain in region of kidneys, urine scant, *Apis mellifica* 3.
Cutting, burning pains in the urethra on urinating, urine often passed in drops, *Cantharis* 3.
Strangury, *Cantharis* 3.
Sticking pains, worse on pressure, *Berberis vulgaris* θ, five drops.

Laryngitis.—Loss of voice, cannot speak above a whisper, *Causticum* 6.
In beginning, with fever, dry skin, restlessness, *Aconite* 3.
Hard, dry, barking cough, *Spongia* 3. Follows well afer *Aconite*.
Œdema glottidis, *Apis mellifica* 3.
Loose, rattling, mucous cough, *Hepar sulphuris* 6.
Chronic, with hoarseness, and viscid, gray, jelly-like mucus, easily hawked up, *Argentum met.* 6x.

Leucorrhœa.—Burning, milky, in those of a scrofulous heredity, *Calcarea carbonica* 6.

Acrid, creamy, in blondes, *Pulsatilla* 3.

Acrid, creamy, in brunettes, *Sepia* 3.

Always tired and weak, *Aletris farinosa* 1.

Watery, excoriating, yellow, *Lilium tigrinum* 3.

Very excoriating and acrid, itching with debility, *Kreosotum* 6.

Greenish, foul, fig warts, *Nitric acid* 6.

Albuminous, white, bland, no pain, *Borax* 3.

Acute, congested, *Belladonna* 3.

With prolapsus; atonic states, *Helonias dioica* θ, five drops. A good general remedy. "It seemed really possessed of great curative virtues."—Hughes.

In inveterate cases, *Alumina* 30.

Liver.—Perhaps the nearest to a "specific" in all liver ills is *Chelidonium majus* θ, in one to five drop doses, twice a day. This is Burnett's great "organ remedy" for liver diseases.

Nausea, pain, vomiting, enlargement of both liver and spleen, *Carduus marianus* θ, five drops in water, morning and evening.

Where patient is troubled with cold hands and is nervous or easily frightened, *Calendula* θ, five-drop doses once a day.

"The seat of action of *Chelone glabra* is in the left lobe of the liver and its line of action is in the direction of the navel, bladder and uterus."—Burnett. θ, five-drop doses, twice a day.

Stitches and pressure in liver; pains as if bruised; worse from motion, *Ranunculus* 3.

Dull, grinding pain, worse when lying on right side; dull pain in region of gall-bladder, *Dioscorea* 3.

Cancer of the liver, *Cholesterine* 3x, three times a day.

Bilious debility, *Ferrum picricum* 6.

"Lazy livers of the city," *Leptandra* 3x.

Jaundice and liver ills in infants, *Myrica cerifera* 3.

For the pain caused by the passing of biliary calculi, *Calcarea carbonica* 30. "In this it has for me quite superseded *Chloroform* and the hot bath."—Hughes.

China 15., in decreasing doses, will prevent the recurrence of gall-stone colic.

Black, fœtid, tarry stool, *Leptandra Virginica* 1x.

Congested liver, stitching pains, *Bryonia* 3.

Patient cannot lie on right side, enlarged liver, clay-colored stools, *Mercurius vivus* 6.

Natrum sulphuricum 6x is the "tissue remedy" for all liver ills, according to Schuessler.

Locomotor Ataxia.—In early stages of the disease, *Secale cornutum* 3.

If traceable to syphilis, *Nitric acid* 6.

Easily exhausted, *Picric acid* 3.

Trembling hands, atrophy of optic nerve, incoördination, *Argentum nitricum* 6.

Lumbago.—The best remedy for lumbago, and pain and stiffness in the small of the back is *Rhus tox.* 3. If *Rhus* fails to give relief in a day or two change to *Berberis vul.* θ in five-drop doses.

If brought on by exposure to dry, cold, *Aconite* 3.

If with the muscular pains there are restlessness and sleeplessness, *Actæa rac.* 3.

If chronic, *Sulphur* 30.

Lungs—Pneumonia.—As an early remedy there is none better than *Aconite* for the chill, fever and restlessness.

For the stage when painful breathing, cough and rust-colored sputum appear, *Bryonia* 3.

Foul, purulent exudation, hectic fever, *Hepar sulphuris* 6.

Typhoid pneumonia, or when case deviates, *Phosphorus* 3.

Cough, troublesome dreams, *Hyoscyamus* 3.

Kafka claimed that *Iodum* 3., every hour, would arrest hepatization.

Red streak down the centre of the tongue, *Veratrum viride* 3.

Kali muriaticum 6x and *Ferrum phosphoricum* 6x, in alternation, constitute the Schuessler treatment for all cases.

For cough remaining after other symptoms have cleared up or for delayed resolution, *Sulphur* 6.

When paralysis is threatened, *Cuprum met.* 12x.

Patient blue and cold, *Carbo veg.* 30.

Congestion of the Lungs.—*Aconite* 3. will cut short the majority of cases.

Pulmonary edema when it develops during the course of other diseases, *Phosphorus* 3.

Short, rapid breathing; suffocation threatened, *Tartar emetic* 3.

Drowsiness marked, *Ammonium carb.* 6.

Lips blue, mucous râles, *Ipecacuanha* 3.

Spitting of blood. If case be of a tuberculous nature, *Bacillinum* 30th or 100th once a week in connection with the indicated remedy.

Cough, violent; blood, bright red, *Acalypha Indica* 3.

No cough, bubbling sensation, with profuse discharge of red blood, *Ipecacuanha* 3.

Dark blood, may be clotted, *Hamamelis* 1x.

For weakness following great loss of blood, *China* 3.

Red, frothy blood, *Millefolium* 1x.

Fear of death, mental anguish, very marked, *Aconite* 3.

Occurring in low fevers, *Phosphorus* 3.

Marasmus.—Open fontanelles, poorly developed teeth, weak spine, emaciation, *Calcarea phos.* 12x.

Scrawny neck and greasy skin, *Natrum mur.* 30.

Acid, sour, head sweats, feet damp, *Calcarea carb.* 6.

Great hunger, yet patient rapidly emaciates, *Iodine* 6.

Child resembles an old person, dwarfish, sluggish, *Baryta carb.* 6.

Wrinkled, cold, dry, with a tuberculous heredity, *Abrotanum* 3.

Sulphur 30. is a good intercurrent remedy.

Measles.—For the fever, restlessness, etc., *Aconite* 3. is the remedy and will often be all that is needed in uncomplicated cases.

When eruption appears, *Pulsatilla* 3.

Skin dusky, eruption retarded, *Sulphur* 6.

Black measles, hæmorrhagic, malignant, great prostration, *Arsenicum* 6.

Oozing of watery blood that will not coagulate, *Crotalus* 6.

Recession, with convulsions, *Cuprum metallicum* 6.

Dry, painful cough, *Bryonia* 3.

Gelsemium 3. is strongly indicated where patient shows great apathy.

When a case of measles breaks out in a family give the unaffected members three doses of *Pulsatilla* 3., as a prophylactic.

Meningitis.—The consensus of opinion seems to point to *Cicuta virosa* 3., as the remedy for cerebro-spinal meningitis, or spotted fever, spasms, head drawn back, twitches, dilated pupils.

Helleborus nig. 3. is a remedy for paralytic stage.

Intense congestion, body hot, pain in head, violent headache, *Belladonna* 3.

Screams when moved, *Bryonia* 3.

Cases marked with languor or drowsiness, *Gelsemium* 3. A remedy very often needed.

Typhoid-like condition, dry, brown tongue, *Rhus tox.* 3.

With violent convulsions, *Cuprum met.* 6.

Trembling feet, *Zincum metallicum* 6.

Shrill cries in sleep, *Apis mellifica* 3.

If patient has tuberculous diathesis give *Bacillinum* 30., or 100., once a week, as an intercurrent.

Menstruation.—Too soon, when there is a tendency towards shorter intervals, *Calcarea carb.* 6.

Too soon and flow lasts too long; cramps, *Nux vom.* 3x.

Painful; colicky pains with bearing down feeling and tenderness of the abdomen, *Chamomilla* 3.

Painful; if occurring in persons of mild and

timid temperament and flow is scanty, black and clotted, *Pulsatilla* 3. See "Dysmenorrhœa."

Too profuse; attended with weakness; black lumps, *China* 1.

Simple menorrhagia, bright red discharge, *Ipecac.* 3.

Flow excessive, preceded and followed by discharge of non-menstrual blood, *Ustilago* 3.

Retarded or suppressed menstruation, especially when it is the result of a chill, *Pulsatilla* 3. See also "Women."

Mental.—Wild, terrifying hallucinations; sees snakes, rats, etc., is at times very loquacious; TERROR, the ruling notes for *Stramonium* 6.

Fears loss of understanding, nervous, *Argentum nit.* 30.

Fears to be left alone, *Arsenicum alb.* 30.

Senile dementia, loss of memory, confused, weak, *Baryta carb.* 30.

Night terrors, *Kali phos.* 12x.

Sees faces, etc., in the shades of twilight, *Phosphorus* 30.

Fear of death; fear of crowd, *fear* in general, *Aconite* 3.

Lewdness, lasciviousness, uncovers person, or sees ghosts, *Hyoscyamus* 3.

Melancholia, with suicidal thoughts, or tendencies, can scarcely refrain from suicide, *Aurum metallicum* 6.

Grief, silent, oppressive, melancholia, *Ignatia* 3.

Illusions, visions, minutes seem years, hears voices, *Cannabis Indica* 1.

Mania, with nymphomania, *Platina* 30.

Thinks his body is in pieces, *Baptisia* 3.

Loss of memory. To prevent stage fright, *Anacardium orientale* 3.

Well known places and things seem strange, *Glonoinum* 3.

Mania and jealousy from sexual causes in women, *Apis mellifica* 3.

Mental and nervous breakdown, men cry like women, *Kali phos.* 6x.

Mumps.—For initial fever, restlessness, etc., *Aconite* 3.

When disease has developed, *Mercurius vivus* 6.

If testicles become involved, *Pulsatilla* 3.

If delirium, or sharp pains occur, extending to the ear, *Belladonna* 3.

If suppuration threatens, *Sulphur* 6.

Neuralgia.—Brought on by exposure to dry cold, or draughts, *Aconite* 3.

Pain marked with burning sensation, *Arsenicum* 6.

Where pain seems to almost drive the patient frantic, *Chamomilla* 3. or 30.

Where pain is borne patiently, or with great weeping, *Ignatia* 3.

Pain settles over left eye or rages in upper jaw, *Spigelia* 3., or θ. *Spigelia* θ is a good general remedy in neuralgia.

Neuralgia of the rectum, *Belladonna* 3.

Neuralgia starting from the eyes, *Ruta graveolens* 3.

Neuralgia in stumps—amputation, *Kalmia lat.* 3.

Magnesia phos. 6x, in hot water, is a fine remedy for all neuralgic pains.

Gaultheria θ, tablets, five a dose, will often cure neuralgia of the stómach and inflammatory rheumatism.

Plantago maj. θ in hot water is very useful in almost all kinds of neuralgia as a local application.

Neurasthenia.—Nervous conditions and impaired memory from voluntary or involuntary emission of semen, *Anacardium orientale* 3.

Nervous breakdown, emaciation, sallow skin, easily frightened, *Argentum nitricum* 6.

Great irritability, especially in children, *Chamomilla* 3.

Nervous, hysterical, sleepless, *Ambra grisea* 30.

Jerking and twitching of the muscles, *Hyoscyamus* 1.

Walking in sleep, *Bryonia* 3.

Cannot keep fingers still, *Kali bromatum* 6.

Fidgeting feet, *Zincum met.* 6.

Brain fag in business men, mental inactivity, slight exertion brings on exhaustion, *Kali phos.* 6x.

Always hurried, querrulous, laughs one moment cries the next, *Ignatia* 3.

Fainting spells, *Moschus* 6.

Melancholy, associated with religion, *Platina* 30.

Nose-bleed.—Bleeding from nose, the best remedy is *Millefolium* 3.

With throbbing headache, *Belladonna* 3.

To stop ordinary nose-bleed snuff up *Hamamelis* extract.

Paralysis.—Facial paralysis, *Causticum* 6.

Paralysis of the lower limbs, *Rhus tox.* 3.

Wrist drop, *Plumbum* 6.

Brought on by exposure to cold, *Aconite* 3.

From degenerative process, *Phosphorus* 3.

Paralysis of single parts, *Gelsemium* 3.

Paralysis in the aged, *Conium maculatum* 3.

Diphtheritic, *Causticum* 6. or *Nux vomica* 3.

From suppressed eruption, *Sulphur* 6.

Paralysis agitans, *Tarantula Cubensis* 6.

Cerebral paralysis, congestion, *Belladonna* 3.; coma, dusky face, *Opium* 3.; from traumatic causes, *Arnica* 3. If patient recovers, give several doses of *Sulphur* 30.

Peritonitis.—Originating in exposure to cold; fever, restlessness, rapid pulse, *Aconite* 3.

Violent throbbing of carotids; tense, swollen abdomen, *Belladonna* 3.

Splitting headache, worse from motion; thirst, *Bryonia* 3., secondary stage.

Suppurative stage, *Mercurius* 6.

With typhoid tendency, *Rhus tox.* 3.

Urine scanty, *Apis mel.* 3.; or bloody, *Cantharis* 3.

Anguish, thirst, vomiting, *Arsenicum* 6.

Excessive distension of abdomen, *Terebinthina* 3.

In convalescence give *Sulphur* 6.

Pleurisy.—The chief remedy for this disease is *Bryonia* 3., indicated by sharp, stitching pains, aggravated by motion.

In first stages, for chill and following fever, *Aconite* 3.

In period of exhaustion, *Sulphur* 6.

Purulent exudation, or when complicated with bronchitis, *Hepar sulph.* 6.

Scanty urine, dyspnœa and palpitation, *Cantharis* 3.

For exudation, *Apis mel.* 3.

If case becomes purulent, *Carbo veg.* 6.

Sulphur 30. is a good intercurrent remedy in all cases that do not run a normal course.

Pleurodynia.—The chief remedy for myalgia, intercostal neuralgia or pleurodynia is *Ranunculus bulbosus* 3., it is especially indicated where the pain is very intense.

Where pain is worse on the right side, *Cimicifuga* 3.

Where pain is stitching and aggravated by motion, *Bryonia* 3.

Arnica 3., where cause is traceable to overexertion or accidents.

Pneumonia.—(See Lungs.)

Prostate Gland.—For enlarged prostate, *Sabal serrulata* θ, five-drop doses.

Cannot pass urine without aid of a catheter, *Solidago virga-aurea* θ, five-drop doses.

Acute inflammation, *Thuja* 3.

Quinsy.—In first onset, flushed face, throbbing carotids, headache, the throat a bright red, *Belladonna* 3.

Common forms of sore throat with pronounced tendency to glandular enlargements; worse on the right side, *Mercurius jod. fl.* 3x.

Ulcerated sore throat with much glandular swelling, worse on the left side, *Merc. jod. rub.* 3x.

Where the pains are of a stinging nature; red, swollen, dry throat; no thirst, *Apis mel.* 3.

When abscess begins to form, *Hepar sulphur.* 6.

To prevent the recurrence of the disease, *Baryta carbonica* 6., one dose a day for a week.

Rectum.—Neuralgia of the rectum, *Belladonna* 3.

Intense itching, *Ratanhia* 3. and *Ratanhia suppositories*. The same treatment also applies to anal fissure and diseased conditions generally.

Prolapse, *Ferrum phos.* 6x, or *Nux vomica* 3.

Fissure, *Graphites* 6., or *Sulphur* 6.

Rheumatism.—Rheumatism brought on by exposure to cold and wet, pain drives patient to motion and motion relieves, *Rhus tox.* 3.

Where patient wants to remain perfectly quiet, motion aggravates the pains; acute, attacking some special part, *Bryonia* 3.

Constant pain, stiffness, pain impels to constant motion, drawing pain, *Causticum* 6.

In cases where there is much fever, hot, dry skin and restlessness, *Aconite* 3. This is especially true if the attack was brought on by exposure to dry, cold weather or winds.

Cases that are worse from warmth, worse at night in bed, and sweat much, *Mercurius vivus* 6.

Pain wanders from place to place, *Pulsatilla* 3.

When pains appear whenever the weather changes to dampness, *Calcarea phosphorica* 6x.

The chronic cold variety, *Kali bichromicum* 3.

In ankle or wrist, *Ruta graveolens* 3.

Viola odorata 3. "curiously cures rheumatism in upper parts of the body when on the *right* side."—Hughes.

THERAPEUTICS. 103

When the small joints of the hands and feet are affected, *Caulophyllum* 3.

Rheumatism in knees or elbows, lance-like pain, but no inflammation or swelling, *Argentum metallicum* 6.

Tearing pains, superficial in warm weather, deeper in cold weather, worse at night, *Colchicum* 3.

Syphilitic, *Phytolacca* 3.

Gonorrhœal, *Natrum sulph.* 6x.

Red, swollen, intolerable to the touch, *Benzoic acid* 6x.

Aching in muscles, *Cimicifuga* 3.

Worst cases of inflammatory rheumatism, *Gaultheria* θ, five-drop doses. Use one drop tablets.

All long standing cases of this disease will be benefitted by occasional doses of *Sulphur* 30.

Chronic joint affections, especially of the knees, connected with urinary difficulties, *Berberis vulg.* θ.

Ringworm.—In all cases of ringworm, in addition to local measures, one dose a week of *Bacillinum* 30. or 100.

If there is much head sweat, *Calcarea carb.* 30.

Sulphur 30. is also a useful remedy where there are flushes of heat.

Sepia 3. is also useful in this disease.

Scarlet Fever.—*Belladonna* 3. is the remedy

that cures what is known as the Sydenham variety of this disease, the smooth, bright red species. The same remedy, administered in time, will check the spread of the disease to other members of the family.

For the malignant variety, dark, purplish, livid throat, stupor, the worst form, *Ailanthus* 1x.

Miliary rash, swollen throat, urine scanty, dropsical tendencies, *Apis mellifica* 3.

Retrocession of eruption, *Cuprum acet.* 6.

When the skin of body looks like a boiled lobster give intercurrent doses of *Sulphur* 6.

Sciatica.—With numbness of limbs or tingling sensation, *Aconite* 3.

Worse on sitting down, better on arising and not felt when lying down, *Ammonium muriaticum* 6x.

One of the best remedies for this disease is *Colocynthis* 3., pain comes and goes suddenly.

Brought on by exposure to cold and wet, *Rhus tox.* 3.

Markedly relieved by warmth, *Arsenicum* 6.

Sulphur 6. is a good intercurrent in all longstanding cases.

Scrofula.—In this disease *Sulphur* 6. is probably the most useful remedy; coarse skin, dirty, shriveled.

In cases where there is head sweat and cold, clammy hands and feet, chalky look, *Calcarea carb.* 6.

Tendency to boils and suppuration, *Silicea* 30.

Sticky eruptions, enlarged glands, cracked skin, *Graphites* 6.

If there is a suspicion of a tuberculous taint, give *Bacillinum* 30. once a week.

The tissue, or Schuessler, remedy for scrofula is *Calcarea phos.* 6x.

Skin.—Hot, dry, feverish, *Aconite* 3.

Red and itching, as from frost-bite, *Agaricus* 3.

Red spots, burning, itching; wheals, puffy under eyes, *Apis mellifica* 3.

Dry, scaly, bran-like scales, *Arsenic.* 6.

Blotches from which exudes a sticky ooze, eczema, angry scars, *Graphites* 6.

Every slight injury suppurates, itching rash in bends of knees and elbows, *Hepar sulph.* 6.

Red eruptions or blotches, which itch intensely, at times making patient scratch until place is raw, *Mezereum* 3.

Itching and burning eruptions, vesicular herpes, eczema, *Rhus tox.* 3.

Brown spots, humid tetter, skin yellow, yellow saddle on nose, *Sepia* 3.

For excessive suppuration from any cause, *Silicea* 30.

Coarse, dirty skin; patient has an aversion to washing; black pores, comedones; with these in any skin disease, *Sulphur* 6.

Nettle rash, hives, prickly heat, *Urtica urens* IX.

Proud flesh, ulcers, splinter-like pains, *Nitric acid* 6.

Fig-warts, *Thuja* 30.

For crops of warts, *Ferrum picricum* 3x.

"Greasy" skin, *Natrum mur.* 30.

Pimples, *Berberis vulg.* θ.

Sleep.—Mind excessively active and all senses too alert, *Coffea cruda* 30.

Sleep prevented by starting, as if frightened, *Veratrum album* 30.

Awakes early and unable to go to sleep again, *Sulphur* 30.

Unconquerable desire to sleep after dinner, awakening much exhausted, *Lycopodium* 30.

Always awakes from sleep *worse, Lachesis* 30.

Sleep prevented by persistent startings, *Ignatia* 30.

Wants to sleep, but fears to; as soon as the eyes close sensation as of a hideous dream, *Cocculus Indicus* 30.

Sleep prevented by restlessness, cannot lie still, *Aconite* 30.

Sleeplessness, prevented by worries over business or other affairs, *Ambra grisea* 30.

In teething children, *Chamomilla* 30.; this failing try *Belladonna* 30.

THERAPEUTICS.

It is generally admitted that in remedies for sleeplessness, etc., higher potencies are better.

One exception to this rule, however, is a remedy which has acquired much reputation without being a narcotic, *Passiflora incarnata* θ, in doses of from five to sixty drops.

Small-pox.—The remedy that, perhaps, has been longest in use in homœopathic treatment of small-pox is *Variolinum* 30. This nosode is said not only to prevent the disease, but when it is developed causes it to run a short and easy course.

Among the other remedies *Tartar emetic* 6. heads the list.

Thuja 30. has also been successfully employed.

For the hæmorrhagic cases *Arsenicum* 6. is the remedy.

In "black small-pox" *Crotalus* 6. is recommended.

Rhus tox. 3. is the remedy where the disease assumes a typhoid character; dry, cracked tongue, sordes and wandering mind.

Sulphur 1x is claimed to be not only a preventive against the disease, but a good remedy with which to conclude the case, clearing up any possible complications.

For "homœopathic vaccination" *Variolinum* has been recognized by the Supreme Court of

Iowa as a legal vaccination when given internally. It is oftenest used in the 30x.

Spermatorrhœa—Emissions.—Where emissions are exceedingly frequent and weakening, great physical debility, little or no power of erection, *Phosphoric acid* 3.

Passive losses during sleep, vertigo on rising in the morning, *Selenium* 30.

Where there are frequent, tense, painful erections, with "furious" emissions, *Picric acid* 30.

With night sweats, *Calcarea carb.* 6.

For ill effects of masturbation, dark rings about the eyes, sallow complexion, sunken cheeks, gloomy, *Staphisagria* 3.

Exhausting emissions with no erections, impotence, *Lycopodium* 30.

Excitable yet impotent, *Agnus castus* 3x.

Hypochondriasis, *Conium maculatum* 3.

Spleen.—*Ceanothus Americana* θ, in five-drop doses, was regarded as the specific "organ remedy" by Burnett for practically all the diseases of the spleen, and the truth of this has been confirmed by other physicians.

Prescribe any other remedy indicated in connection with the *Ceanothus*.

Summer Complaint.—(See Cholera Infantum.)

Sunstroke.—For immediate and remote effects, *Glonoinum* 6.

For headache that may return every summer,

from the effects of a stroke, *Natrum carbonicum* 6.

Stomach.—Ills arising from green fruit, vegetables, ice, or ice cream, *Arsenicum* 6.

From indigestible food, feeling of a stone in stomach, bitter, bilious, waterbrash, headache, *Bryonia* 3.

Feeling of weakness in pit of stomach, *Ignatia* 3.

Gastric catarrh, acidity, heartburn; a little food, a few mouthfuls, causes satiety, *Lycopodium* 30.

The slightest deviation of diet causes distress, *Natrum carbonicum* 6.

Burning in stomach, *Arsenicum* 6.

As soon as water becomes warm in the stomach it is vomited, *Phosphorus* 3.

Acidity, *Natrum phosphoricum* 6x.

Sick stomach, nausea, *Ipecac.* 3.

Vomiting dark blood, *Hamamelis* 1x.

Vomiting bright red blood, *Ipecacuanha* 3.

Pain in stomach relieved by eating, but which returns shortly, *Anacardium orient.* 3.

Gastric ulcer, *Argentum nitricum* 6. Olive oil *pure* is one of the best remedies for gastric ulcer, cancer of the stomach, and for many other ills of that organ.

Syphilis.—The chief remedy for all primary cases is *Mercurius vivus* 6.

Where the case is a very severe one, ulcerative, acute, buboes, *Mercurius corrosivus* 6.

In advanced cases where ulcers have eaten in, ulcerous throat, bleeding gums, foul odor from mouth; or in cases that have received too much and too strong doses of medicine, *Nitric acid* 6x.

In cases where the bones are affected, nose eaten into; ozæna, patient very gloomy and despondent, *Aurum metallicum* 6.

The above remedies are the chief ones in the homœopathic treatment of this disease. The following may be useful as intercurrents, as called for by their several symptoms:

For the nightly bone pains, *Mezereum* 6.

Excessive suppuration, *Silicea* 30.

Discharge very corroding and burning pains, *Arsenicum* 6.

Copper colored spots, eruptions on scalp, around chin, itching eruptions, *Sulphur* 6.

Fig warts or cauliflower excrescences and for the headache of syphilis, *Thuja* 30.

Sore throat, not ulcerated, *Phytolacca decandra* 3.

Teeth.—Toothache in old and decayed teeth, or in several at once, the whole row, *Mercurius vivus* 6.

Toothache following filling the teeth, *Arnica* 3.

Burning, throbbing, worse at night, hot gums, *Belladonna* 3.

Toothache, relieved by holding cold water in the mouth, *Coffea cruda* 3.

Brought on by cold water or air, *Calcarea carb.* 6.

Teeth feel sore and too long, *Rhus tox.* 3.

"Jumping" toothache, *Sulphur* 6.

Teeth decay early and turn black, *Kreosotum* 3.

Neuralgic pain in teeth, *Magnesia phosphorica* 6x.

Of *Plantago major* Hughes says "it will cure seven-tenths of the cases of toothache," it should be given where there are no clear indications for another remedy.

Enamel rough, *Calcarea fluorica* 6x.

Ulcerated teeth, *Mercurius vivus* 6.

Abscess, *Silicea* 30.

Tetanus.—The best general remedy for lockjaw is *Hypericum perforatum* in the 1x or mother tincture. When the preliminary shooting pains appear this remedy will abort the disease in many cases and cure many more fully developed. Tetanus generally follows injuries to nerve and "*Hypericum* is to laceration and torn wounds what *Arnica* is to blows and contusions." Whether this remedy is curative in tetanus following other causes than nerve injuries, as, for instance, vaccination, is an open question. If there is a feeling of soreness, *Arnica* 3. will aid.

Acid hydrocyanicum 6. has cured the disease. *Nux vomica, Cicuta virosa* and *Stramonium* have all been used with more or less success.

Throat.—The best remedy for ordinary "sore throat"—inflammation of the throat—is *Belladonna*. The symptoms calling for this remedy are burning and dryness.

Mercurius is the remedy for catarrhal sore throat, body and limbs ache, profuse perspiration, worse in damp weather. Much saliva which one is forced to swallow though the act is painful.

Aconite is especially indicated when there is much fever, great restlessness and fear.

Nitric acid is called for when there is splinter-like pain; also when there is a history of syphilis.

Lycopodium is more especially called for in chronic cases, worse about 4 P. M., with fan-like motion of nostrils.

Phytolacca is indicated in bluish colored throat, with a feeling of scraping rawness and dryness. This remedy, like *Belladonna*, has a strong affinity for the throat, but has less fever, but more aching.

Hepar sulph. is called for when a sore throat goes on to suppuration.

Lachesis.—This remedy is called for when there is swelling of the submaxillary and salivary glands, and also extreme sensitiveness to touch, and patient cannot bear anything binding about the throat.

Mercurius corrosivus.—Intense inflammation and ulceration with threatened suffocation.

Typhoid Fever.—Feels tired, very tired, dreads motion, body feels sore, frontal headache. A remedy for early stages when limbs feel heavy, lassitude, headache, loss of appetite, etc., *Bryonia* 3. A remedy that may abort the disease, but is of no use when diarrhœa sets in.

Drowsy, going to sleep while talking, dark tongue, besotted looking face, mental depression, bed feels too hard, thinks body is scattered about bed, sordes on teeth, exhalations and evacuations very fœtid, *Baptisia* 1x or 3.

Ulcerative stage, putrid decomposition, triangular red tip to tongue, muttering, may refuse medicine, nose-bleed, restlessness, possibly involuntary stools, and trembling chin, *Rhus tox.* 3.

Bruised, sore feeling, indifference, ecchymoses, petechiæ, involuntary stool, and discharge of urine, dropping of jaw, *Arnica* 3.

Case has run a long time, patient profoundly prostrated yet restless, intense fever, everything worse after midnight, very red tongue, thirst, picks at bed clothes, *Arsenicum* 6.

In *extremis*, cold, pulseless, discharges horribly offensive, Hippocratic face, *Carbo veg.* 30.

In cases marked by little or no thirst, dry, hot skin, dry, cracked, trembling, swollen tongue, *Apis mellifica* 3.

Where there are marked cerebral symptoms, *Belladonna* 3.

Hæmorrhages of dark blood, *Hamamelis* 1x.

Delirium, *Hyoscyamus* 3.

Abdomen tympanitic, constipation, rumbling in bowels, patient sinks down in bed, unconscious, *Lycopodium* 30.

Where paralysis of the brain is threatened, or occurs, *Zincum metallicum* 6.

Excessive urination in convalescence, *Causticum* 6.

Low forms marked by very foul evacuations, *Muriatic acid* 3.

Urinary Disorders.—Urine hot, passed in drops, persistent, or violent urging, *Cantharis* 3.

Sudden retention of urine, *Mercurius cor.* 6.

Very painful urination, *Belladonna* 3.

Incontinence of urine in children, *Cina* 3. or five-drop doses of *Rhus aromatica* θ. *Nux vomica* 3. has also cured many cases of enuresis.

Brick dust sediment in urine, *Lycopodium* 30.

Urine smoky, turbid, coffee-ground sediment, or bloody, *Terebinthina* 3.

Vile odor, smells like that of a cat, *Benzoic acid* 3. or *Cina* 3.

Paralytic conditions, last few drops are slow in passing, *Causticum* 6.

Clay-like sediment adhering to sides of chamber-pot, *Sepia* 3.

Dribbling of urine, *Stramonium* 3.

Old men must use catheter to pass urine, *Solidago virga-aurea* θ, five drops.

Much mucus and pus in urine, *Chimaphila umbellata* θ, five drops.

Cannot retain urine, *Ferrum phos.* 12x.

Bad effects of long retention of urine, *Causticum* 6.

Spurting of urine when coughing, *Causticum* 3.

Constant calls to urinate, *Apis mellifica* 3.

Frequent urging at night in old people, *Causticum* 3.

Full of uric acid, *Thlaspi bursa pastoris* θ, ten drops in wineglassful of water. (Rademacher.)

Vaccinosis.—A word coined by Burnett for the ills acute or remote following vaccination. For these, *Thuja* 30. is the remedy.

Voice.—Hoarseness, with inflammation of the throat, or with cold in the head, *Belladonna* 3.

Hoarseness and rawness in the larynx. Clergyman's sore throat, *Arum triph.* 6.

From simple catarrh, *Causticum* 6.

Whooping Cough.—When cough runs into convulsions, *Cuprum metallicum* 6.

Where the whoop is very marked and clear, *Mephitis* 6.

Severe paroxysms, changing color of face, *Magnesia phosphorica* 6x.

In cases not marked by any severe symptoms, *Drosera rotundifolia* 1x.

"Minute gun" variety, or smothering, *Corallium rubrum* 6.

With tenacious, stringy mucus, *Coccus cacti* 3.

Rattling of mucus, white tongue, *Tartar emetic* 6.

To prevent the spread of the disease give *Drosera* 1x to the other children, or to those liable to contract the disease.

Wounds.—For blows, concussions or any heavy fall, etc., *Arnica* 3. internally and *Arnica* tincture, one part to twenty of water externally.

For cuts, bleeding wounds, lacerations, torn or jagged wounds, wherever the flesh bleeds from other causes than severe concussions or blows, *Calendula* θ, or, better, *Succus calendulæ* (the pure juice) applied externally. "Pus cannot live in the presence of *Calendula.*"

For any fever or inflammation following hurts of any kind, or operations, give *Aconite* 3. internally.

For mashed fingers, or punctured wounds

caused by needles or nails or anything penetrating, *Hypericum perforatum.* Dress externally with the pure tincture and give 3d decimal internally. This remedy is especially useful in wounds from "toy pistols," or where lockjaw may follow. The remedy for nerve hurts.

Where hurts heal slowly and suppurate, *Hepar sulphur.* 6.

Blood poisoning from cuts, dissecting, putrid meat, disease or any cause resulting in the condition generally known as "blood poisoning," *Lachesis* 6.

Gangrene, from any cause, *Lachesis* 6.

Scalds with steam, or hot water, bathe with a strong solution of common washing soda and internally give *Apis mel.* 3. Later anoint wound with cerate of *Echinacea.*

To promote union of broken bones, *Symphytum* 3., internally, and the tincture externally.

Women.—Scanty menstrual flow; leucorrhœa, chlorotic blondes; better in open and cold air, *Pulsatilla* 3.

Yellow complexion, yellow saddle on nose, dark rings about the eyes, colicky pains; scant, or too profuse menstruation; leucorrhœa; bearing down pains; brunettes, or dark complexioned, *Sepia* 3.

Menstrual difficulties associated with rheumatism, *Cimicifuga racemosa* 3.

Menstruation of bright red blood; inflammation, slight jar causes pain, throbbing, *Belladonna* 3.

Profuse menstruation, irregular, cold damp feet, anæmic, appetite for unnatural things, milky leucorrhœa, cough, *Calcarea carb.* 30.

Cramp-like pains extending to bowels and rectum. Menstrual colic, *Caulophyllum* 1x.

Dirty, greasy skin, *Natrum mur.* 30.

Always better from coolness and the open air, *Pulsatilla* 3.

Soreness, weight, aching in womb; vaginitis, *Helonias dioica* θ. "The best of uterine tonics." Five-drop doses in water.

Menses suppressed from bathing, *Antimonium crud.* 6.

Suppressed menses, patient hysterical, nervous, *Senecio aureus* 1x.

Nerve fag in connection with sexual diseases, *Zincum valerianate* 6.

Dr. J. C. Burnett, in that most valuable little work, *Organ Diseases of Women*, introduces *Fraxinus Americana* θ as an individual remedy in hypertrophy of the uterus, and claims to have by its means saved many a woman from a surgical operation. Dose, five drops of tincture three times a day.

Another useful remedy is *Nymphæa odorata*, in the form of suppository, in cases of prolapsus uteri, vaginitis and ulcerations. It has been termed "the vegetable curette."

Probably the two remedies most often indicated in menstrual disorders are *Sepia* and *Pulsatilla*, the former for the dark complexioned and the latter for blondes, is a good, broad distinction.

Worms.—Sickly, pale, rings around the eyes, gnashing of teeth, child picks its nose, canine hunger, *Cina* 30., the chief homœopathic remedy.

Stannum met. 6. is another remedy that has done good work in freeing the system from lumbrici and ascarides.

Yellow Fever.—For the preliminary onset of fever, *Aconite* 3.

If onset is dull, apathetic, patient dull, *Gelsemium* 3.

Nausea, vomiting, burning, thirst, *Arsenicum* 6.

In the "black vomit" type, *Crotalus horridus* 6.

In collapse, *Carbo veg.* 30. This remedy is also a prophylactic.

PART III.

MATERIA MEDICA.

Materia Medica (the knowledge of what conditions a drug will cause in a healthy human being) is the corner-stone of Homœopathy. "Therapeutics" are merely convenient indications—finger posts—showing the general direction. You must match the patient's symptoms from *similar* in the materia medica. The following materia medica is made up of some of the land marks of each drug, which should be studied in its totality in the larger works. Still this abridged materia medica will guide any one to a cure in the average run of cases.

Abrotanum.

(Southernwood. Tincture from fresh leaves.)

Marasmus, with a tuberculous heredity, or tuberculosis developed. Moist.

Weak, hectic fever, shrunken legs; eats well, but emaciates.

Flabby skin.

Dose: 3d potency.

Aconite.

(Monkshood. Tincture from fresh plant, including the root.)

In all typical *Aconite* cases, *mental distress, anxiety, restlessness* and *fear* are very prominent. Also the preceding chill followed by *fever*, with hot, dry skin.

Effects of *fright*.

Ailments originating in exposure to *dry cold*, or to checked perspiration caused by draughts.

In *inflammation* from any cause.

Cases preceded by *chill*, followed by *fever;* incipient coryza, stiff neck, lumbago, etc.

Menstrual disorders brought on by sudden chill or exposure to dry cold.

The first remedy in *croup*, and in all *acute diseases*, preceded by chill or fever.

Neuralgia and rheumatism with *numbness* or *tingling* of limbs.

The action of this remedy is not of long duration. It will abort many acute diseases, but if the disease progresses it is no longer useful. *Aconite* is the greatest of fever remedies when the fever is not that resulting from septic states.

Dose: 1x to 30th potency.

Æsculus hippocastanum.

(Horse chestnut. Tincture from hulled nuts.)

The action of this remedy is principally on the lower bowel.

Protruding, purple, *bleeding* piles, or non-bleeding with *backache*. Feeling as though rectum were full of sticks; torpid liver, backache, etc.

Liver ills associated with hæmorrhoids.

Dose: 3d to 6th potency.

Agaricus muscarius.

(Poison mushroom. Tincture from fresh fungus.)

Twitching of eyelids, of various muscles, *involuntary jerking* of various muscles; tremors; itching; chorea; St. Vitus' dance.

Red, *burning, itching* of ears, hands and feet, as if frost bitten; chilblains. Involuntary movements.

Tumultuous heart action of inveterate tea and coffee drinkers and of smokers.

Dose: 3d, 6th or 30th potency.

Agnus castus.

(Chaste tree. Tincture from fresh berries.)

The central feature of this drug is sadness and *loss of sexual power*. Premature ageing from abuse of sexual organs.

Impotence following gonorrhœa.

Dose; 3x to 6x potency.

Aletris farinosa.

(Star grass. Tincture from the fresh roots.)

Used when there is an anæmic and relaxed

condition, especially of the female organism and the patient is always tired and weak. Prolapsus, leucorrhœa, extreme constipation. Chlorotic females.

Dose: Tincture to 3d potency is used.

Allium cepa.

(Tincture of the fresh ripe onion.)

Nearly every one knows the effect of raw onions on the eyes and nose; both water profusely, burn and smart, and are acrid. It is just this sort of *"cold"* or *coryza similar* to this that this drug will cure.

Dose: 3d, 30th or 200th potency.

Aloe.

(Tincture from inspissated juice.)

Venous congestion. *"Loss of confidence in sphincter ani"* is a classical homœopathic indication; afraid to pass wind or urine for fear fæces will escape.

Hæmorrhoids like grapes; covered with mucus.

Mucous stools; rectum sore after stool. Constipation; painful, but useless urging to stool; burning in anus. A combination of lumbago headache and piles.

Dose: 3d to 30th potency.

Alumen.

(Common alum. Triturated with sugar of milk.)

The chief use of this remedy is in *lead poisoning, printer's colic,* and constipation; no ability to expel stool. Paralytic weakness, dryness and contraction are the keynotes.

Dose: 6th to 30th potency, preferably the latter.

Alumina.

(Oxide of Aluminum. Triturated with milk sugar.)

The keynote to this drug is *"dryness;"* dry mucous menbranes, dry catarrh, dry intestinal tract, dry skin, etc. Lack of vital heat, prematurely old, sluggish.

Hard stools, rectum inactive, with peculiar feature that even when stools are soft they are *difficult of expulsion.*

For girls who eat slate pencils, chalk, etc.

Heavy dragginess of *lower limbs.*

Sexual weakness in those of advanced years. Prostatic discharges, involuntary emissions while straining at stool. Urine difficult to start flowing.

Dose: 6th to 30th or 200th potencies.

Ambra grisea.

(Ambergris. Triturated with sugar of milk.)

This is distinctly a *nervous* or *hysterical* remedy. Patients always in a *hurry.*

Sleeplessness in thin, scrawny, nervous men and women. Old persons who *forget* the simplest things. Worn out. Parts of body *"go to sleep."* Nervous, spasmodic, hollow coughs, choking when phlegm comes up.

Dose: 6th to 30th potency.

Ammonium carbonicum.

(Carbonate of Ammonium. Triturated with sugar of milk.)

This is especially adapted for stout persons who lead a sedentary life. The mucous membrane of the respiratory tract is especially affected, and the persons are very sensitive to cold air and have a great aversion to water; cannot bear to touch it. Congestive fullness and raw feeling of the chest with slate-colored mucus. Drowsiness; patients are tired and weary.

Dose: 3x to 6x potency.

Anacardium orientale.

(Marking-nut Tree. Tincture from crushed seeds.)

Mentally there is a *desire to curse and swear.* Hypochondria. Fixed ideas. A feeling as of having two wills. Hears voices. *Loss of memory.* A dose taken before appearing in public prevents *stage fright.*

Nervous dyspepsia. *Dyspepsia* that is *relieved* by eating, but soon returns as food is digested. Headache relieved by eating, but returning soon.

Feeling as of a *plug* in various parts; of a *band* around the body.

Eczema resembling *Rhus* poisoning; itching, burning.

Dose: 6th to 30th potency.

Antimonium crudum.

(A crude ter-sulphuret of antimony. Triturated with sugar of milk.)

Worse from *cold water*, internally or externally. Characterized by coated *milk-white* tongue. Extreme *irritability* and *fretfulness*. Child does not want to be touched or looked at. *Worse* from heat of sun. Cough *worse* coming into a *warm room*.

Stomach disorders, no appetite, heartburn, nausea. *Indigestion* from sweet things. Eructations tasting of food.

Nostrils cracked and scurfy. Small boils or pimples around mouth or nose.

Child *vomits milk* in curds.

Rheumatism where *soles of feet are very tender;* heels sore. Nails split, brittle and out of shape.

Alternating *diarrhœa* and *constipation* in elderly persons.

Piles, with mucus like white of eggs.
Eruptions around *genitals.*
Dose: 3d to 30th potency.

Antimonium tartaricum.

(Tartar emetic. Triturated with sugar of milk.)

Great accumulation of rattling *phlegm on the chest,* with inability to raise it. Old persons cannot cough up the phlegm. Drowsiness, debility and sweat.

Pneumonia, catarrhal croup, bronchitis. Any respiratory affection marked with great accumulation of mucus, which is not easily coughed up. Short breath. Sits up to breathe.

Child wakes *gasping* and *choking* from accumulation of phlegm.

Cholera morbus with nausea, vomiting.

Great *drowsiness* and generally pale face.

When eruptions in scarlet fever, measles, etc., *do not come out.*

Pustular eruptions. Small-pox.

Dose: 3d to 30th potency.

("Tartar Emetic Syrup," as prepared by homoeopathic pharmacists, is an excellent form for dispensing this drug.)

Apis mellifica.

(Made from the honey bee. Live bees are shaken in a bottle until thoroughly angry and then alcohol poured on them. APIUM VIRUS: The stings are extracted and triturated with sugar of milk. Either preparation may be used.)

General characteristics are *puffy swellings, no thirst; drowsiness, worse from heat; stinging pain in any part of the body,* relieved by cold applications, bagging under the eyes.

Acute, *swollen throat,* inside red; *diphtheria; scarlet fever,* with very rough rash; *nettle rash,* stinging and burning.

Legs and feet waxy and swollen; dropsy; waxy skin.

Urine scanty.

Sudden *starting* and *screaming* of children during sleep; brain diseases, meningitis.

Stinging pain and inflammation of *eyes* or *eye-lids;* serous exudation.

Erysipelatous inflammation in various parts; swollen, hot.

Inflammation of kidneys during or following eruptive diseases.

Dose: 3x to 30th potency.

Apocynum cannabinum.

(Canadian hemp. Tincture or decoction of fresh root. Sometimes improperly called Indian hemp.)

The chief use of this drug (largely empirical) is in the treatment of *dropsy.* It is prepared as a tincture and as a decoction, and the latter preparation is the one chiefly used, giving by far the best results. *Apocynum cannabinum decoction* in teaspoonful doses twice a day has gained green laurels in the cure of uncomplicated dropsy and hydrocephalus.

It also has a reputation for putting *alcoholics* on their feet—the trembling, "on-their-last-legs" cases. *Excessive vomiting.* In the latter, twenty- or thirty-drop doses.

Dose (tincture) : Ten drops.

Argentum metallicum.

(Pure precipitated silver, triturated with sugar of milk.)

Increased secretion of mucous membranes.

Chronic laryngitis with hoarseness and *viscid*, gray, jelly-like mucus, easily hawked up.

Swelling of glands, especially of testicles, with pain as if crushed.

Heart frequent, spasmodic, *painless twitching* of *cardiac muscles.*

Bad effects from abuse of Mercury.

Soreness of joints, arthralgia. Numbness of limbs.

Vertigo, as if intoxicated; vertigo on looking at running water.

Chronic gleet.

Dose: 6x to 15x potency.

Argentum nitricum.

(Nitrate of silver, dissolved in distilled water and potentized.)

Headache deep in the brain, hemicrania, vertigo, debility and trembling. Head feels enormously enlarged. Afraid to be alone. Photophobia. Threatened paralysis.

Paralysis from spinal affections.

Melancholia, mentally depressed, trembling of whole body.

Purulent ophthalmia (30th potency).

Intense craving for sugar or sweets.

Thick, tough, *tenacious* mucus in the throat.

Catarrh of smokers.

Gastritis of drunkards.

Diarrhœa *caused* by excitement.

Purulent gonorrhœa or leucorrhœa.

Indicated in children who seem like dried up old men or women.

Dose: 6th, 30th or 200th potencies.

Arnica montana.

(Leopard's bane. Tincture from fresh plant including the roots.)

The great indication for this drug in disease is a *sore, bruised feeling* as though the body had been beaten or pounded. Of great use, internally (and externally, one part of the tincture to twenty of water) in all blows, falls and concussions.

Heart troubles of *athletes*.
Crops of boils.
Typhoid, head hot but body cold; putrid stools.
Bed feels too hard. Bedsores.
In any illness where *nose* is abnormally *cold*.
Internally to prevent *suppuration* or ecchymoses in injuries.
Affections following *injuries*, concussions.
Toothache after filling.
Gout with fear that some one will approach affected part.
Dose: (Internally) 3d to 30th potency.

Arsenicum album.

(Arsenious acid. Triturated with sugar of milk.)

The great keynotes to *Arsenicum* are *malignity, restlessness, anguish, burning* and *periodicity*. *Great prostration*, worse from cold and rest; thirst. *Nightly aggravations.* Better from heat. Blood gets dark, malignant. "What *Aconite* is to simple fever *Arsenicum* is to its malignant form." "No remedy is more restless than this one in later stages."

Thin, burning, acrid discharges in any diseases.

Pains like *hot needles,* neuralgic.
Skin *dry* and *scaly, dandruff.*
Burning lachrymation from eyes; *photophobia,* ciliary neuralgia.
Watery, *burning,* excoriating discharges from nose, *grippe, colds.*
Burning pain in the teeth and gums.
Lips so dry that patient licks them.
Ailments from taking *cold things*—ice water, ice cream, green vegetables, etc.
Hæmorrhoids that burn like fire.
Urine, in passing, burns like fire.
Burning sciatica, better from warmth.
Cholera, with intense burning in stomach, yet may be cold outside.
A prophylactic against effects of the bites of animals.
Cancer, with burning pain.
Intermittent fever, violent thirst during sweat.
Dose: 3x, 6th, 30th or higher.

Arum triphyllum.

(Jack-in-the-pulpit. Indian turnip. Tincture of the fresh root.)

Eruption, like scarlet rash, with itching, skin peels afterward. Acridity characterises this drug.

Hoarseness and rawness in the larynx; the control over the voice is lost; an excellent remedy in clergyman's sore throat. Acrid condition of the nose—hay fever, coryza.

Dose: 6th to 30th potency, and should not be repeated often.

Arundo Mauritianica.

(Reed. Tincture from root sprouts.)

The provings of this remedy present an almost perfect picture of *hay fever*—violent sneezing, nose red and raw looking, constantly blowing it, itching, burning; eyes inflamed, lachrymation. The remedy is very efficacious in *hay fever*.

Dose: 3x potency.

Aurum metallicum.

(Pure precipitated gold. Triturated with sugar of milk.)

A deep acting remedy, much used by Arabian physicians of old.

The prominent, guiding mental symptom is *melancholia* with *suicidal tendencies.* Disgust for life.

Especially useful in worst stages of *syphilis* when disease has attacked the bones. *Caries of bones.* Bone pains. Foul breath.

Combined effects of syphilis and overdosing of mercury, etc.

Syphilitic ophthalmia.
Red knobby nose. *Ozæna, very foul.*
Chronic orchitis.
Complaints marked by coming on only in winter.
Dose: 6x to 30th potency.

Asafœtida.

(Devil's dung. Tincture of the gum resin.)

This is most useful in a nervous, hysterical, scrofulous temperament; the symptoms are worse from nervous excitement. Hysteria of the flatulent order. Sensation of a ball rising from the stomach to the throat; obliging frequent swallowing. *Patient full of wind.*

Asthmatic state of the respiratory organs.

Periosteal inflammations and ulcerations. Caries. Rickets.

Dose: 2x to 30th potencies used.

Bacillinum.

(The difference between the homœopathic *Bacillinum* and the old school *Tuberculinum* is that *Bacillinum* is made direct from the bacilli of tuberculosis and the *Tuberculinum* from the cultivated bacilli. The homœopathic preparation is triturated to the 6x with sugar of milk and then from the 6x make a dilution.)

The best information for the use of the remedy is to be found in Dr. J. C. Burnett's *New Cure for Consumption With Its Own Virus*. The nosode has never been more than tentatively proved, but the meagre provings go to show its striking *similarity* to *consumption*. Very useful in *ringworm*.

In every case where there is a suspicion of *tuberculous*, or *consumptive heredity*, this drug, with other remedies, will work wonders. In incipient stages of tuberculosis it will often radically cure the disease, and in advanced stages will give more relief than any other remedy.

Dose: 30th, 100th and 200th. *Not oftener than once a week.*

Baptisia.

(Wild Indigo. Tincture from the fresh roots.)

The chief sphere of this drug is in *typhoid fever*, which it will both abort and cure.

The *Baptisia* patient has in the beginning chilliness, aching pains, muscular soreness, and nervousness. Later, there is drowsiness, the patient falling into a drowse or mentally wandering while answering a question; the face has a besotted, dusky look. Still later may complain of being in pieces, or scattered about the bed. Muttering delirium. Very foul diarrhœa. Livid spots.

Intolerance of pressure. Indescribable sick feeling.

Skin of forehead seems drawn.
Ulcerated gums and mouth.
Diphtheria, patient *can only swallow liquids.* Very offensive breath.
Dose: 1x to 30th potency.

Baryta carbonica.

(Carbonate of barium. Triturated with sugar of milk.)

Defective growth, mentally and physically, children *prematurely aged,* and grown persons *prematurely childish,* are the leading indications for this anti-scrofulous drug.

Premature impotency. Foot sweat.

Paralysis of the aged. Senile dementia. Memory lost. Apoplexy in the aged. Tongue paralysis.

Suppurating tonsils. *Quinsy*—curative and as a prophylactic.

Chronic aphonia in the scrofulous.

Dose: 6x to 30th potency.

Belladonna.

(The deadly nightshade. Tincture from fresh plant.)

This drug is only useful in acute cases, characterized by unnaturally *bright, dilated eyes,* hallucinations, *throbbing,* mania, violent delirium and fever. Hot head. *Jarring* and *light* **aggravate.** Congestion of brain.

Blinding headache, worse from light, or the least jarring, stooping, or lying down. Rush of blood to the head. *Meningitis.*

Scarlet fever, the chief remedy, bright red skin. Sydenham variety.

Acute *inflammation of the ears,* terrific pain.

Erysipelas. Facial neuralgia, comes on like a flash, worse from slightest jar.

Sore throat, bright red, glazed looking, very dry. A great throat remedy.

Boils, carbuncles, toothache, any condition where there is much *throbbing.*

Restless sleep of children, eyes half closed, head hot, twitching, starting.

A wild, red hot remedy.

Dose: 3d to 30th potency.

Benzoic acid.

(Triturated with sugar of milk.)

Recent attacks of *gout, hot, swollen finger-joints, or wrists,* red, swollen, *painful joints,* associated with strong smelling urine, uric acid conditions, is the sphere of this remedy.

Worse in open air and does not want to be uncovered.

Dose: 3x to 6th potency.

Berberis vulgaris.

(Barberry. Tincture of the fresh bark of root.)

This is indicated when there are pains in or radiating from the lumbar region; lumbago; it is therefore useful in renal and vesical troubles, and vesical catarrh. It also has liver symptoms with sticking pains under ribs, which pains go from the liver to the abdomen; bilious colic, gall stone, and colic.

Arthritic and rheumatic complaints connected with urinary or liver troubles.

Dose: Tincture to sixth potency.

Bismuthum.

(Precipitated Subnitrate of Bismuth is triturated with sugar of milk.)

Irritation and catarrhal inflammation of the alimentary canal, especially of the stomach, are the chief indications for this remedy. Frequent eructations and distressing pressure and burning in region of stomach. Slow digestion.

Has the peculiar symptom of aching teeth or gums that are *better* from cold applications.

Dose: 1x to 3x trituration is used.

Borax.

(Triturated with sugar of milk.)

The most pronounced and the best verified indication for this drug is *"fear of downward motion"*—the instant one starts down the stairs, or attempts to lay the child down, or rocks it, it screams and exhibits great fear and disturbance. The same applies to adults, though, of course, they will not scream.

Edges of eyelids inflamed.

Erysipelas, face feels as if it had cobwebs on it.

Sore mouth (aphthæ). (Do not use crude drug.)

Dose: 3d to 6th, or 30th potencies.

Bryonia.

(Wild hops. Tincture from fresh roots.)

This drug corresponds to more symptoms of daily occurrence than any in the Materia Medica. "If I were confined to one drug, I would choose *Bryonia.*" Hughes.

The most marked symptoms are *worse from motion* and *better from presure;* patient lies on painful side, which runs all through the *Bryonia* symptomatology. Good without regard to *name* of disease. Mucous membranes are very *dry*.

Short, quick breathing, pain in chest, must *hold chest* while *coughing;* hot, red face, *rusty* or *bloody sputa, pneumonia,* frequent desire to take long, deep breath.

Frontal *headache, splitting;* bitter eructations, bitter taste, waterbrash, biliousness, pressure in the stomach, feels sore; headache worse from moving eyeballs, bursting, splitting.

Acute rheumatism attacking particular joints or muscles; stiff neck.

Pleurisy, pneumonia, peritonitis, and *constipation.*

Dry mucous membranes, drinks large quantities of water, lips dry, throat dry, tongue dry, dry cough.

Eyeballs very painful, especially on motion.

Very dry catarrh.

Gastric derangements, feeling of a load in the stomach, a stone there.

Liver seems swollen, sore to the touch; coated tongue.

Patient is averse to sitting up, wants to lie quiet and be let alone.

Ills following the sudden advent of hot weather.

Dose: 1x to 30th potency.

Cactus grandiflorus.

(Night-blooming Cereus. Tincture from fresh plant and flowers.)

The great sphere of this remedy is the *heart,* and its characteristic symptom is sensation of constriction of the heart, as if an iron band prevented its normal movement. *Angina pectoris,* cardiac dropsy, hypertrophy of heart, palpitation of heart, myocarditis, dyspepsia with heart complications.

Dose: θ to 6x.

Caladium seguinum.

(American Arum. Tincture of the whole fresh plant.)

This remedy has a marked action on the genital organs. Frequent nocturnal emissions, sexual desire with relaxed penis. It is one of the best remedies for pruritus vulvæ, impotence. Masturbation. Itching, burning rash, alternating with asthma.

Dose: 3d to 30th potency is used.

Calcarea carbonica.

(Trituration of the pure white, middle layer of the oyster shell. Calcarea ostrearum. Carbonate of lime.)

The leading indications for this great antipsoric remedy are *scrofula, sweating head; cold, damp feet, large abdomen, big head* and small neck (in children), sour vomiting, obesity, flabby, short breath, torpid; pale, chalky skin, *curvature of bones* or spine, *fontanelles open, marasmus,* easily takes cold.

Joints swollen, with no inflammation.

Chronic headache with vertigo; headaches of school children, scrofulous. Headache with cold hands and feet.

Scrofulous inflammation of ears, polypi; purulent discharges, bleeding.

Ulcerations in nose, *polypi.*

Acid stomach, *dyspepsia,* hot or warm food disagrees; craving for unnatural things, slate pencils, chalk, etc., etc.

Diarrhœa of undigested stool.

Young girls, delayed menses, palpitation, anæmia, leucorrhœa, milk white. Aching in vagina. Milk of nursing woman disagrees with child.

All ills are *worse from ascending,* from exertion and dampness. Better in dry warmth.

Big appetite yet patient emaciates.

Scabby eruptions.

Hectic fever, cold extremities, *night sweats.*

Fat, flabby, scrofulous, cold, sweaty, hectic, etc., etc., calls for this great remedy.

Very efficacious in internal *tumors* which grow slowly for years.

Dose: 6th, 30th and 200th potencies.

Calcarea fluorica.

(Crystals of fluorspar. Triturated with sugar of milk.)

This is one of the "Schuessler," "tissue"

or "biochemic remedies;" also homœopathic, as are *Natrum mur., Silicea,* etc. Whether the action is biochemic, or homœopathic, is immaterial. The action is there, and it is the same whether administered on homœopathic, or biochemic indications, between which there is little if any distinction.

Hard, lumpy growths, bone tumors, tumors discharging *bone splinters, enlarged joints,* chalky deposits, *glandular swellings, fistulous* openings.

Cataract of the eyes.

Varicose veins, enlarged veins, hæmorrhoids.

Hardened wax in the ears.

Rhagades, chapped hands.

Dose: 3x to 12x potency.

Calcarea phosphorica.

(Precipitated phosphate of lime. Calcium phosphate. Triturated with sugar of milk.)

This is another of the Schuessler remedies and its indications are: *Bone diseases, rickets, tuberculosis, kidney* affections, *leucorrhœa,* "whites," *chlorosis, nightsweats, scrofula,* fistula, emaciation in children, teeth decay rapidly, dyspepsia, *rheumatism in damp weather,* and, broadly, is always indicated in *white exudations.*

Hydrocephalus, diseased tonsils in strumous, scrofulous patients.

Every cold causes rheumatic pains in joints.

To aid in the *uniting of broken bones,* and in delayed dentition.

For children of defective nutrition, emaciated, flabby abdomen, large heads, weak neck and spine, vomits milk, *worse in damp weather,* malnutrition, headaches of school girls.

Dose: 3x to 12x potency.

Calendula officinalis.

(Marigold. Tincture of flowering plant.)

The chief use of this remedy is as an external application to promote the *rapid healing* of all manner of *bleeding, chafed, torn, jagged* or *raw wounds.* "*Pus cannot live in its presence,*" and it is nature's royal and genuine antiseptic.

Also very valuable as an external dressing for *cancer, ulcers* and *tumors.* Also, in cerate form, for all cases of chapped hands.

The best form in which to use this remedy is in what is known as *Succus Calendulæ, i. e.,* the pure juice with only enough alcohol added to preserve it from fermentation.

Use freely as it is not poisonous.

Camphora.

(Tincture made by dissolving gum camphor in alcohol.)

The keynote to this drug is *collapse with coldness.*

It is especially indicated in the first onset of *Asiatic cholera,* and Dr. Rubini (whence "Rubini pellets of camphor") treated over five hundred cases of that disease in Naples with this drug alone without losing a single case.

Camphora has the peculiar symptom that the patient does not want to be covered.

Icy coldness of whole body.

Dose: The Rubini pellets in Asiatic cholera, otherwise 3d to 30th potency.

Cannabis Indica.

(Hashish, Indian hemp. Tincture prepared from dried herb-tops.)

The most prominent symptoms of this drug are mental—minutes seem ages, ideas crowd the mind, things seem in huge perspective. Loss of speech from mental causes, words will not come. *Catalepsy.* Incoherent talk. Laughs or cries at trifles. *Spectral illusions.* Clairvoyance.

Backache, constant, with no amelioration. Backache from sexual abuse.

Dose: 1x to 30th potency.

Cannabis sativa.

(American hemp. Tincture prepared from fresh tops.)

There is essentially but little difference between this drug and the *Cannabis Indica* save that the former is more potent.

This drug has a reputation in the cure of uncomplicated *gonorrhœa* where the urethra is very sensitive to the touch. *Mercurius cor.* follows well.

It is also useful in *opacity of the cornea* and in *cataract*—white film on eyeball.

Dose: 1x to 30th potency.

Cantharis.

(Spanish fly. Tincture of dried flies reduced to powder.)

Violent *pains in bladder;* urging to urinate; cutting, burning, *scalding* pains in urethra; *urine passed drop by drop* or none will pass. Strangury. Constant urging to urinate. *Urine bloody. Cystitis. Nephritis.*

Pains generally that feel as if "on fire"—any part of the body.

Furious sexual desire, amounting to mania. Amorous excitement. *Priapism. Nymphomania.*

Gonorrhœa, chordee with intense sexual excitement.
Acute inflammation of eyes, biting, smarting pain. Erysipelas.
Throat feels as if on fire.
Pleurisy, burning pain.
Vesicular, burning, eruptions.
Dose: 3d to 30th potency.

Capsicum.

(Red pepper. Tincture from dried peppers.)

Pains of a burning character, yet accompanied with shivering, chilliness, or shuddering.

Atonic dyspepsia of hard drinkers; *morning vomiting;* allays intense craving for liquor.

Intermittent fever where the sweat comes with the fever. Excessive thirst, but shivering from drinking. Pain in back and limbs; chill begins in the back.

Chronic diarrhœa—blood and matter (pus) discharged from the ear.

Weak stomachs.
Dose: 1x to 6th potency.

Carbo vegetabilis.

(Vegetable charcoal. Triturated with sugar of milk.)

Flatulence, belching, acidity, heartburn; oppression after each meal. *Dyspepsia.*

Hæmorrhage in low type of disease; *dark blood.* Recurring nose-bleed.

Blueness, *coldness,* cold breath, cold tongue, collapse, in any disease. Cold from feet to knees.

Chronic hoarseness; *bronchitis.*

Patient "wants to be fanned"—in any disease, a leading symptom.

For ailing ones who date their debility from "ever since I had the ——," whatever disease, or event, it may have been.

This drug does not act well in the low potencies.

Dose: 6th to 30th, or 200th potency.

Carduus Marianus.

(St. Mary's Thistle. Tincture prepared from the seeds.)

The chief use of this remedy is in the cure of *varicose veins* and in enlarged liver with "sternal patches," brownish eruptions. Soreness in region of liver.

One of Rademacher's remedies.

Dose: 5 drops of the θ.

Caulophyllum.

(Blue cohosh. Tincture from the fresh roots.)

A *woman's remedy,* acting on uterus and small joints.

Dysmenorrhœa, uterine *cramps;* severe labor *pains;* bearing down pains. Lochia protracted.

"Internal shivering."

Finger joints, ankles or toes, in pregnant women, swell and are sore.

Discoloration of face from menstrual disorders.

Dose: θ to 30th potency.

Causticum.

(Burnt lime and fused bisulphate of potash, distilled; a preparation peculiar to Homœopathy. Tincture.)

The urinary symptoms of this drug are very prominent. *Urine spurts involuntarily* when coughing, sneezing, walking, etc. Urine passes so easily that he is almost unconscious of its escape; or in *paralytic conditions of the bladder* urine is slowly expelled or even retained. *Enuresis.*

A remedy for ill effects of long retention of urine, as when one has no opportunity to urinate.

Very hoarse. *Loss of voice.*

Cough where one cannot raise the mucus; compelled to swallow it.

Paralysis of single parts. Paralysis after diphtheria or other diseases. Paralytic conditions generally.

Sickly yellow face (not jaundiced). Facial neuralgia at every change of weather.

Dose: 6th to 30th potency.

Cedron.

(Simaba Cedron. Tincture from the seeds.)

The keynote to this drug, in *malarial fevers* and neuralgias, in which it is chiefly used, is the *clock-like regularity* of the attacks. In cases of this sort when attacks can be foretold almost to the minute *Cedron* is possibly the remedy.

It also seems to be specially adapted to persons with chill and fever, returning from warm climates.

Dose: 1x to 6th potency.

Chamomilla.

(German chamomile. Tincture prepared from fresh flowering plant.)

The *Chamomilla* patient (often a child but not always so) is marked by a *cross, spiteful, peevish, moaning, whining mood,* wants things and then fretfully refuses them, pushes them away. Always complaining. Is also (and this accounts for the disposition) very sensitive to pain. When patient is quiet though suffering this remedy will do no good.

Fretful, cross, *teething children.* When there is *one cheek red and the other pale* the remedy is writ large. Head sweat.

Rheumatism, neuralgias, labor pains, etc., that "drive patient wild."

A peculiar yet verified symptom is the *giving way of the ankles* every afternoon.

Insomnia in fretful children.

Green, slimy, mucous *diarrhœa* in infants and young children. Wind colic.

Pain with marked numbness.

Ills following anger.

Rheumatism in adults that drive them to get up and walk about.

Dose: 6th, 15th or 30th potencies.

Chelidonium majus.

(Celandine. Tincture prepared from fresh plant.)

This is the "organ remedy" in all *liver disease,* jaundice, gallstones, hepatitis, and one of its chief symptoms is a *pain under the right shoulder-blade.* But whether this is in evidence or not, give it a trial in liver ailments.

Enlarged liver. Biliousness. Yellow skin. Yellow tongue. Lethargy. Yellow diarrhœa. Pneumonia, where there is liver disease.

Dose: 5 drops of θ to 6x. The tincture is most effective.

Chimaphila umbellata.

(Pipsissewa. Tincture from entire fresh plant.)

The only known use for this remedy is in *catarrh of the bladder*, with turbid, ropy urine with pus or mucus in it; may be bloody.
Useful in prostatic troubles.
Dose: Five drops θ.

Chininum arsenicosum.

(Arsenite of Quinine. Triturated with sugar of milk.)

The chief use for this drug is in *uncomplicated diarrhœa*, in which it is quickly curative.

It is also useful in cases where the patient is *tired and weary*, prostrated and weak.
Dose: 3x to 6x trituration.

Cicuta virosa.

(Water hemlock. Tincture from fresh root.)

A remedy for *violent convulsions*, especially where the patient bends backward, opisthotonos; frightful distortions.

Is curative in *cerebro-spinal meningitis*, especially the malignant variety.

Infantile convulsions where child *bends back*.

Convulsions from injuries, from wounds.

Cramp in neck throwing the head back.

Dose: 3x to 30th potency.

Cimicifuga racemosa.

(Black snake root. Tincture from the fresh root.)

Reflex *neuralgias,* dependent on ovarian and uterine troubles; also *rheumatism* in those same troubles; rheumatism of the belly muscles.
Puerperal mania, talks much; suspicious.
Woman's headache, associated with uterine and ovarian troubles; cough; spinal irritation.
Neuralgias of ovaries and uterus.
Aching eyes from prolonged use and consequent headache.
Dose: 1x to 6th potency.

Cina.

(Wormseed. Tincture from dried flowers.)

Picking and boring at the nose with the fingers, itching, itching anus, canine hunger, irritable temper, screams, jerking head, rings about the eyes, grinding teeth during sleep are the leading symptoms pointing to this medicine. Especially useful in worm cases in children.

Like all homœopathic remedies it may be called for in many other diseases if the symptoms of patient indicate, even in typhoid.

Dose: 1st, 6th or 30th potencies.

Cinchona—China.

(Calisaya Bark. Tincture of dried bark.)

Weakness and debility from loss of fluids, semen, blood, over-nursing, diarrhœa, suppuration or sweating (diuresis).

Dark rings around sunken eyes; sallow, pale face; night sweats, rapid emaciation, roaring in the ears.

It is the great antihectic.

Painless diarrhœa.

Headaches of anæmics, pulsating in temples.

Constant satiety, belching, dyspepsia, coldness of the stomach.

Affections that are worse every other day.

In *intermittent fever* the chill, fever and sweat are distinctly marked with intervals; great thirst precedes chill and sometimes headache; profuse sweat, very debilitating; roaring in the ears.

This drug has the curious symptom that a slight touch aggravates, but hard, firm pressure relieves.

Dose: 1x to 30th potency.

Cocculus Indicus.

(Indian cockle. Tincture from dried fruit.)

Vomiting and sickness caused by riding in cars, carriages, ships—by riding.

Great repugnance to food.

Wants to sleep, but on closing eyes is assailed by frightful sensation as of a hideous dream.

Headache in back of head and nape of neck.

Great vertigo usually accompanies *Cocculus* ills. Whirling vertigo.

Nausea and vomiting are also frequent concomitants.

For pure, uncomplicated dysmenorrhœa.

Intermittent fever in which these general symptoms are more or less in evidence.

Dose: 3x to 30th potency.

Clematis erecta.

(Virgin's bower. Tincture of the fresh leaves and stems.)

Moist, itching eruptions, worse from washing in cold water. Painful swelling and induration of glands. Painful swelling of testicles, especially the right, also inguinal glands.

Dose: 1x to 6th dilution.

Coccus cacti.

(Cochineal. Tincture from the dried insects.)

A remedy for coughs and *whooping cough,* where paroxysm ends in vomiting *clear, stringy and ropy mucus. Kali bichromicum* has stringy mucus also, but it is yellow.

In any disease where this *clear, white, stringy mucus* is in evidence this remedy may prove useful.

Dose: 1x to 6th potency.

Coffea cruda.

(A tincture prepared from the unroasted green Mocha coffee beans.)

The leading use of this drug is in *sleeplessness*, where the mind is unnaturally active and crowded with ideas and thoughts; great mental activity. Nervousness with unnatural exaltation of all the senses.

Headache caused by excessive coffee drinking.

Toothache and neuralgias relieved by cold applications.

Dose: 3d, 6th, 30th, or 200th potencies. This drug acts better in the higher potencies.

Colchicum autumnale.

(Meadow saffron. Tincture of the fresh bulb in spring.)

Acts on muscles, bones and joints. There is always great prostration. The parts are red, hot and swollen. Tearing pains, worse in the evening and at night and from touch. Anasarca. Hydrothorax. Gout. Rheumatism. Inflammation of digestive tract; nausea and loathing at the thought of food. Autumn dysentery.

Dose: 3d to 30th potency.

Collinsonia Canadensis.

(Stone root. Tincture from the fresh roots.)

A marked sense of *constriction in any or all the orifices of the body* is the leading indication for this drug. Especially useful in obstinate *constipation* and flatulence in connection with protruding *hæmorrhoids*. It is well to insert *Collinsonia suppositories* when the remedy is administered for hæmorrhoids.

Dose: θ to 3d potency.

Colocynthis.

(Bitter cucumber. Tincture prepared from pulp of dried fruit freed from outer rind and seeds.)

Colic and sciatica are the spheres of this remedy. The colic is very severe, causing the patient to bend double, or to press the abdomen against something to relieve the pain. The *Colocynth* pains are relieved by pressure. Uterine colic. Sciatica—all of a neuralgic nature and cramp-like.

Dose: 3d, 6th, or 30th potency.

Conium maculatum.

(Poison Hemlock. Tincture from the whole flowering plant.)

The first proving of this drug is described by Plato in the death of Socrates. It was a good proving, showing the *ascending paralysis* it produces.

A marked symptom is vertigo when turning over in bed. Whether standing, sitting or lying down patient turns his head sidewise.

Losing use of legs. *Locomotor ataxia.* Limbs feel heavy, weary, almost paralyzed.

Ophthalmia, where photophobia is peculiarly intense; strumous patients.

Cancers and *tumors* following injuries or slight blows, or injuries on the breast, etc. Glands feel painful.

Sexual weakness, *emissions* on touch of the other sex, or even sight.

Dose: 1st, 6th, 30th or 200th potencies.

Corallium rubrum.

(Red coral. Trituration with sugar of milk.)

Terrific paroxysms of coughing closely following each other. *Whooping cough.* Barking, "minute gun" cough.

Post-nasal catarrh.

Chancre; flat, coral red ulcers on glans; yellowish discharge.

Dose: 6th to 30th potency.

Crocus sativa.

(Saffron. Tincture from the dried stigmata.)

Useful for hæmorrhages that are black and stringy. Metrorrhagia.

Brain irritation, congestion and hysterical mania (vacillating, ill humor, then lively; strong desire to sing, laugh and jest). Chorea.

Sensation as if something were alive and moving in the abdomen.

Dose: Tincture to 30th attenuation is used.

Crotalus horridus.

(Venom of the rattlesnake. Triturated with milk sugar.)

Putrescence and *bleeding* in fevers. Low, septic states; watery blood.

Oozing of *dark blood* which does not clot or coagulate.

Bloody sweat.

Blood from every outlet of the body.

Nose-bleed in the senile.

Diphtheria, very malignant, *oozing of blood*.

Hæmorrhagic measles.

Malignant *yellow fever,* black vomit.

A very yellow skin is characteristic.

Dose: 6th to 30th potency.

Croton tiglium.

(One part of Croton oil to 99 of alcohol makes the θ.)

Watery, yellow, *choleraic diarrhœa*, gushing out as from a hydrant.

Small red blotches on thighs, body, or around genitals, with intolerable itching.

Eczema with intolerable itching. *Herpes zoster.*

Dose: 6th to 30th potency.

Cuprum metallicum.

(Precipitated copper. Triturated with sugar of milk.)

Cramps and *spasms* are the leading features of *Cuprum*—cramps in fingers, in toes, in feet, in calves, in stomach, in cholera. Especially indicated in *Asiatic cholera* when cramps appear, face blue, cold sweat, etc.

Epilepsy, spasms beginning at fingers or toes; *chorea, convulsions,* meningitis, cerebrospinal meningitis.

Paralysis of hands or arm; paralysis of tongue. *Paralysis* generally.

Copper is an almost sure prophylactic against Asiatic cholera.

Dose: 6x to 30th potency.

Digitalis purpurea.

(Fox glove. Tincture from fresh leaves of uncultivated plant in second year of growth.)

A very slow pulse directs attention to this drug; or very irregular, fluttering or intermittent. Faintness, feels as if dying, cyanosis, difficult respiration, fluttering heart, sudden sinking, breathless on least exertion, inclination to take a deep breath, sadness, all point to this drug.

Sharp pains about the heart.

Dropsies from heart disease, urine scanty and dark.

Dose: 1x to 3x potency.

Dioscorea villosa.

(Wild yam, colic root. Tincture from fresh roots.)

Cramp-like pains, *colic,* call for this remedy and the guide to them is that the patient straightens out, or bends backward, in contradistinction to *Colocynth,* which causes patient to bend forward or double up. Flatulent, wind colics.

Dose: 1x to 6x potency.

Drosera rotundifolia.

(Sundew. Tincture from fresh flowering plant.)

Cough is the leader for this remedy. A cough that comes on while lying down. *Whooping cough.* Tough mucus. Bloody sputum. Has some repute in phthisis.

Dose: 1x to 30th potency.

Dulcamara.

(Bitter sweet. Tincture from green stems and leaves of plant before flowering.)

The great modality of this remedy is for ills that are *worse from cold, wet weather* and sudden change from warm to cold weather—pains in back, diarrhœa, stiff neck, limbs sore, *rheumatism,* stiffness and lameness, headache, neuralgia, cough, urticaria, eruptions, *catarrhal complaints,* and anything brought on or aggravated by cold, damp weather.

Echinacea.

(Purple cone flower. Tincture from the fresh roots.)

The use of this splendid remedy is almost purely empirical, yet its sphere of action has been so often confirmed that it is entitled to a place among the polychrests. The keynote to its use is *septic states*—bad blood. Indicated in boils, tumors, carbuncles, old ulcers, ozæna, foul leucorrhœa, abscesses, cerebro-spinal meningitis, puerperal scepticæmia, diphtheria, typhoid, gangrene, eczema, sepsis, scrofulous ophthalmia,

small-pox, bites of animals; in fact, in any depraved state of the blood this remedy will do good work in connection with the indicated remedy.
Dose: 5 to 20 drops of θ.

Epiphegus.

(Beech drop. Tincture from the fresh plant.)

The range of this remedy is in *sick headache* brought on by any deviation from the even tenor of her way—shopping—any unusual excitement.
Dose: 1x to 3d potency.

Erigeron.

(Canada fleabane. Tincture of the whole fresh plant.)

This is chiefly known as a remedy for *hæmorrhoids* and congestions. Hæmorrhages in nearly any part of the body; characterized by the *bright red color*, and increased by the slightest motion of the patient.
Dose: Tincture and lower potencies may be used.

Eucalyptus.

(Blue gum tree. The mother tincture is made from the fresh leaves.)

Headache of a dull congestive character, coryza, sore throat, indigestion, with excessive development of fœtid gas, and fever. Slow digestion is the character.

Influenza. Malarial troubles. Fevers of a relapsing character.

Diuresis and great increase of urea.

Dose: Tincture and lower potencies may be used.

Eupatorium perfoliatum.

("Boneset." Tincture from entire fresh blooming plant.)

The keynote to this drug is found in its common name, boneset, given it because of its great efficacy in relieving the *bone pains* and bone aches of grippe, influenza, intermittents, dengue, break-bone fever; in fact, wherever there are aching bones this remedy is indicated.

Dose: θ to 3d potency.

Euphrasia.

(Eyebright. Tincture from flowering plant, excepting the root.)

The therapeutic range of this drug is in *eyes* and *nose—acrid* lachrymation and *bland* coryza. Catarrhal conjunctivitis; sticky mucus in the eyes.

Dose: θ to 6th potency.

Ferrum phosphoricum.

(Phosphate of iron. Triturated with sugar of milk.)

One of the leading tissue remedies. *Inflammation* is the keynote and guide to *Ferrum phos.*, especially in first stages. Inflammation of eyes, ears, teeth, stomach, joints, wounds, etc.

Pneumonia, pleurisy, inflammatory fevers, headache; all congestive conditions; vertigo.

Rheumatism, lumbago, erysipelas, sore throat, coughs, colds and coryza, in their beginnings.

Hæmorrhages of *bright-red* blood, piles, dysentery, boils, carbuncles and hot swellings; incontinence of urine—wetting the bed; throbbing headache; painful diarrhœa from catching cold.

Dose: 3x to 12x triturations.

Ferrum metallicum.

(Metallic iron. An element.)

This is best adapted for weak, nervous persons, flushing easily, and for delicate chlorotic women.

It is useful in anæmia when there is an appearance of full bloodedness, coldness of the body. Its action is to dilate the blood-vessels.

Irregular distribution of the blood, with headache, nose-bleed, dyspnœa, neuralgia, etc.

Undigested diarrhœa, worse from eating.
Dose: 1st to 30th potency is used.

Gelsemium.

(Yellow Jessamine. Tincture from the thin fresh rootlets.)

Prostration, loss of muscular power, drowsiness, lassitude, dullness, vertigo and *torpidity* point to this remedy.

Paralysis following diphtheria; paralysis of single muscles, of groups of muscles; lose control of muscles; writer's cramp.

Low types of fever; patient dull, wants to be let alone; torpid.

A remedy often indicated in cerebro-spinal meningitis.

Dull, stupid headaches; headache relieved by flow of urine.

Deafness from quinine; of Eustachian tubes.

Little thirst in *Gelsemium* ills.

Seminal weakness, emissions without dreams or erections.

Easily fatigued, cannot use hands, legs give way, trembling, nervous chills.

Dose: 1x to 30th potency.

Glonoine.

(Nitro-glycerine. Tincture prepared by one part of pure drug to nine of 95 per cent. alcohol.)

The sphere of action of this remedy is chiefly in the head, and its remedial action is largely in cases *caused by heat*—heat of the sun or fire. It is the leading remedy in all immediate and remote effects of *sunstroke;* for the headache of printers and all who work under artificial light. The headache is throbbing and pulsating, and very sensitive to the slightest jar.

Patient has a very glowing red face.

Another guiding symptom is that familiar things and places seem strange, "loses his way in well known streets."

Threatening apoplexy.

Dose: 6th to 30th potency. (N. B.—Lower potencies will cause fearful headaches.)

Graphites.

(Black lead. Triturated with sugar of milk.)

The leading indication for this remedy is *oozing; glutinous, sticky eruptions* on any part of the body; where these are in evidence *Graphites* will be the remedy.

Constipation with unusually large, hard stools.

Anus is sore and fissured.

Thick finger-nails that grow out of shape is a keynote to this remedy; also hard, cracked hands.

The remedy covers a large number of cases more or less chronic, eczema, sore eyes, catarrh, erysipelas, throat, gastralgia, liver, enuresis, etc., wherever there is the peculiar moist, sticky eruption.

It is also often the remedy for the ills of fleshy, coarse grained women.

Dose: 6th to 30th potency.

Hamamelis Virginica.

(Witch hazel. Tincture from fresh bark of young twigs and roots. Extract, distilled from twigs when flowering.)

The *Hamamelis* patient is notably without fear, quite unlike the *Aconite* patient, who is generally fearful and dreads that his disease will be fatal.

Bleeding is the keynote to this remedy, dark blood—bleeding piles, bleeding from nose, bleeding from stomach, lungs, orifices of body relaxed; patient is not alarmed at the bleeding, varicose veins. Varicocele.

Dose: θ to 3x, internally. Extract, externally. Suppositories, with remedy internally, for bleeding piles.

Helleborus niger.

(Black hellebore. Tincture from the dried root.)

Useful for weakly, scrofulous children; brain symptoms of dentition.

Dropsical effusions of brain, thorax, peritoneum and cellular tissue; sudden dropsical swellings. Hydrocephalus, meningitis, hydrothorax; anasarca. Sees, hears, tastes imperfectly and general muscular weakness; convulsive twitching of muscles during sleep. Melancholy mania; thumb drawn into palm. Characteristic aggravation from 4 to 8 P. M.
Dose: Tincture to thirtieth dilution is used.

Helonias dioica.

(False unicorn. Tincture from fresh root before flowering.)

Uterine remedy, in *prolapsus, menorrhagia, leucorrhœa* and *atonic states* of the organ, chlorosis. Dragging languor, prostration, backache. Better when engaged in some work or company.

Headache with uterine troubles.

In *Bright's diesease* and kidney trouble it is very efficient—in females.

It is a *uterine tonic* and its prescription, it is asserted, will often be followed by pregnancy.

Dose: Five to ten drops of θ, to 3d potency.

Hepar sulphuris calcareum.

(Impure Calcium sulphide. Triturated with sugar of milk.)

Depressed, irritable frame of mind. Craving for sour things and strong tasting things. *Patient chilly,* cold air makes him cough. *Every little hurt suppurates. Oversensitive,* pimples and sores very painful when touched. Sensitive to pain, touch and cold air.

If pus is threatened this remedy may abort and if formed will promote healing.

Loose, *wheezing, rattling cough,* but mucus is not coughed up.

Nose stopped at every exposure to fresh air.

Feeling as of a splinter in the throat. *Quinsy.* Hypertrophy of tonsils.

Stools, even though soft, and urine passed with difficulty. Never seems able to empty the bladder.

Scrofula and *ulcerations* generally.

Abscesses at root of teeth. Spongy, bleeding gums.

Ailments resulting from overdosing with mercury or iron.

Sensitiveness to cold air, to touch; offensive suppuration and the almost total absence of fevei are the land-marks for this antipsoric.

Dose: 6th to 30th potency.

Hydrastis Canadensis.

(Golden seal. Tincture from fresh roots.)

A combination of *debility, dyspepsia,* and unhealthy mucous membranes indicates this remedy.

Catarrh, yellowish-greenish discharge tinged with blood.

Aphthous sore mouth. Canker in mouth.

Sore throat with hypertrophy of mucous membrane.

Atonic dyspepsia, acidity, torpid liver, earthy skin. Weak, faint, gone feeling in stomach.

Constipation with no other apparent symptoms.

Cancer, lupus and *malignant ulcers.*

Ten drops of the θ in hot water every half hour is a good remedy for gall stones.

Dose: θ to 6th potency.

Hyoscyamus.

(Henbane. Tincture from fresh blooming plant.)

Mania marked by suspicion; loquacious; by lasciviousness; wants to uncover and expose his, or her, person. Senile mania.

Twitching of the muscles very marked.

Dry cough coming on when lying down.

In acute cases, like typhoid, patient picks at

the bed clothes, mutters, eyes staring, but apparently sees nothing.

Convulsions caused by fright.

Dose: 6th to 30th potency.

Hypericum perforatum.

(St. John's wort. Tincture from entire, fresh blooming plant.)

For all injuries to *nerves* or perforated wounds, gunshot wound, toy pistols, etc., especially *tetanus* or *lockjaw* following such injuries.

For torn, lacerated wounds; mashed fingers, splinters, punctures from needles or pointed instruments.

Externally and internally.

Dose: θ to 6x potency.

Ignatia.

(Bean of St. Ignatius. Tincture from the powdered seeds.)

This is a drug of changeable moods. Patient is hilarious and then silent and melancholy. Greatly given to sighing. Hysterical, laughing and crying. Epilepsy from mental causes only.

Silent grief.—The peculiar sinking feeling that comes at the pit of the stomach when some calamity occurs, or at the death of some loved one.

Will relieve undue, silent, brooding grief caused by death in the family.

Headache, sharp and confined to one point.

Prolapsus ani; patient afraid to strain at stool for fear of prolapse.

"Globus hystericus," a feeling as if a lump arose from stomach to the throat.

Intermittent fever—thirst only during chill. Chill relieved by heat. Red face during chill.

Dose: 6th to 30th potency.

Iodium.

(Iodine. Triturated with sugar of milk.)

Irritability of the nervous system. Emaciation with good appetite.

Swelling and induration of glands, mesenteric, inguinal, testicles, prostate, thyroid, etc. It is called for in glandular atrophy, wasting diseases and in scrofulous patients.

It acts on the mucous membrane, especially the respiratory, croupous inflammation, dyspnœa, where there is emaciation.

Dose: The 3d to 30th potencies may be used.

Ipecacuanha.

(Tincture from the dried root.)

Persistent *nausea* and *vomiting*, and *hæmorrhages* of *bright red blood*, are the two great keynotes to the drug.

Fermented, yeasty, green, **watery** and slimy stools. A good remedy for infants.

Menstruation of bright red blood.

In stomach troubles with a clean tongue.

Spasmodic asthma, wheezing dyspnœa, suffocating.

Cough as from inhaling sulphur fumes.

Whooping cough ending in nausea and vomiting.

Intermittent fever (better as a beginning routine remedy than quinine) with persistent nausea in all stages.

Dose: 3d to 30th potency.

Iris versicolor.

(Blue flag. Tincture from fresh root.)

The keynote to this remedy is *sour vomit* and *sick headache,* generally beginning with a blur before the eyes. Also periodic headaches of school teachers, students, etc., which come on when strain of mind is relieved—Saturday or Sunday.

It has been found useful in sciatica of left leg.

Constipation, especially in those subject to headaches, 30th potency.

Dose: 3d to 30th potency.

Kali bichromicum.

(Bichromate of potash. Triturated with sugar of milk.) Whenever the expectoration, or *mucus*, is *tough, stringy* or *rope-like*, there is a strong probability that this remedy is indicated without much regard for the name of the disease.

In diseases of the nose where there are tough, tenacious secretions, "clinkers." Nose stopped. *Perforation of septum.*

Cold, chronic rheumatism.

Diphtheria and croup with *yellow* membranes.

Headache preceded by blindness which passes as headache develops.

Bronchitis and asthma with *stringy mucus.*

A remedy for fat persons very much troubled with phlegm.

Stringy excretions and a general yellow color characterize this remedy.

Face blotched, indigestion, pimples or acne. Pustular eruptions like small-pox.

Syphilitic ulceration of the tongue.

Dyspepsia of beer drinkers.

Dose. 2d to 30th potency.

Kali carbonica.

(Carbonate of potassium. Triturated with sugar of milk.)

The leaders to this drug are: *worse between 3*

and 4 o'clock A. M., *stitching pains,* weak back, sensitive to cold, no perspiration and *bag-like upper eyelids.*

Curative in hip-joint disease.

Anæmic conditions in young girls, white skin, unable to menstruate, constant backache.

Easily frightened, starts at a touch.

"It is rarely that ulcerative pulmonary phthisis can be cured without this antipsoric."—Hahnemann.

Effects of miscarriages and labor at childbirth.

Dose: 3d to 30th potency.

Kali muriaticum.

(Potassium chloride. Triturated with sugar of milk.)

One of the tissue or Schuessler remedies.

In general corresponds to secondary states and follows well after inflammatory conditions; acts chiefly on the mucous membranes. It is also noted for its *grayish-white secretions* or exudations, white or gray coating at back of tongue, white tongue runs through this remedy's sphere. A remedy for chronic states.

Stuffy colds, coughs, hoarseness, dry coryza, mumps, bronchial affections, sick headache, noise in the ear, sores in mouth; diphtheria, first remedy; dyspepsia, indigestion, epilepsy.

Rheumatism, swollen joints the result ot rheumatism, bunions, chilblains, scurfy skin, dandruff, white scales, carbuncles.

Constipation or jaundice with white tongue; gonorrhœa, first remedy.

Deafness from swelling of *Eustachian tubes.* Chronic catarrhal inflammation of middle ear. Sore throat, grayish patches, swollen, ulcerated.

Dose: 3x to 12x trituration.

Kali phosphoricum.

(Phosphate of potash. Triturated with sugar of milk.)

One of the tissue or biochemic remedies.

Kali phos. is the remedy for brain, nerves and blood. *Mental breakdown,* men cry like children; *nervous prostration, neurasthenia, sexual debility, foul conditions of the blood.*

Septic states, typhoid, foul ulcers, all discharges having a cadaverous odor, gangrene; unhealthy, pustulous skin, offensive catarrh and ozæna; foul, offensive diarrhœa, earache, stiff neck.

Hay fever, asthma, eyes red, all paralytic conditions.

Epilepsy, delirium tremens, horrors; a remedy for the aged.

Menstrual colic in the nervous.

Adynamia; decay, mental and physical.
Blood blackish and unhealthy.
Dose; 3x to 12x trituration.

Kali sulphuricum.

(Potassium sulphate. Triturated with sugar of milk.)

One of the tissue or biochemic remedies.

In general the conditions calling for *Kali sulph.* are *worse from warmth* and *better in the cool, open air.* Its discharges are slimy and yellow.

Asthma with rattling mucus and catarrh, yellow discharges, laryngeal catarrh, thin discharges from the ear, fluent coryza, croupy hoarseness.

Catarrh of the stomach.

Headache, better in the open air; dandruff, scaldhead.

Leucorrhœa.

Wandering, shifting pains.

Burning or itching skin, scaly skin, tetter.

Dose: 3x to 12x trituration.

Kalmia latifolia.

(Mountain laurel. Tincture from fresh leaves.)

Rheumatism and neuralgia, rapidly shifting pains, *shooting downward,* involving heart; dyspnœa. Notably all ills are *worse* before a thunderstorm.

Tobacco heart.
Dose: 3d to 6th potency.

Kreosotum.

(Kreosote. Tincture, one part wood tar Creasote dissolved in nine parts of alcohol.)

Profuse and *offensive* secretions. *Leucorrhœa*, very offensive, corroding and yellow.
Early *decay of teeth*—teeth begin to decay almost as soon as they appear.
Gums dark-red, swollen, painful.
Cholera infantum with *incessant vomiting*, from painful dentition.
Sympathetic vomiting, *i. e.*, when from disorder in some other organ than the stomach.
Vomiting of pregnancy.
Characteristic symptom is pain as from red-hot coals. Phthisis and chronic pneumonia.
Dose: 3d to 30th potency.

Lachesis.

(The Bush-master. Venom triturated with sugar of milk.)

Blood poisoning from dissecting wounds; from putrid meat. *Mortification. Gangrene.*
When deposits are slight in *diphtheria*, but *prostration* alarming.
Throat and neck sensitive to touch; *doesn't*

want anything about the throat, not even the bedclothes.

Complaints generally begin on the *left side* and *patient wakes from sleep worse.* Headache. Varicose veins.

Gastralgia, vomiting and trembling of *drunkards.*

Late and worst stages of *peritonitis.*

Worse from touch and pressure.

Dose: 6th to 30th potency.

Ledum palustre.

(Marsh tea. Tincture from the fresh plant.)

Curative, internally, for the effects of insect bites, especially *mosquito bites.*

Rheumatism, beginning in the feet and *traveling up.* Swelling of small joints, toes and fingers. Ankles swollen.

Dose: 1st to 6th potency.

Leptandra.

(Culver's root. Tincture from fresh root.)

Increased secretion in liver and intestinal canal; profuse, black, tarry stool. Jaundice. Biliousness.

Dose: Tincture or low potency is used.

Lilium tigrinum.

(Tiger lily. Tincture of fresh plant in flower.)

Uterine remedy, indicated by a persistent *bearing down pain.*

Hysterical symptoms associated with uterine troubles.

Menses which flow when moving about.

Dose: 3d to 30th potency.

Lobelia inflata.

(Indian tobacco. Tincture of the fresh plant.)

It is useful in *asthma* and *gastric affections* when there is languor with *nausea, vomiting* and *dyspnœa.*

Bad effects of drunkenness.

Cannot hear, taste or smell of tobacco.

Dose: It is used from the tincture to the thirtieth potency.

Lycopodium.

(Club moss. Trituration and tincture.)

Mental, nervous and bodily weakness; sallow skin; no appetite; poor digestion; flatulence, constipation and cold extremities.

Waterbrash. Acidity. Heartburn.

Flatulence, distension, *bloating* of abdomen.

Constipation. Constant fermentation seems to be going on. *Jaundice.*

Sits down *very hungry,* but a few mouthfuls produce a feeling of *satiety.*

Impotence in the elderly; also in young men from masturbation, etc.

Lingering ills following pneumonia.

Very drowsy always after dinner.

Red sand in urine, "brick-dust." Pain in renal region.

Always worse from 4 to 8 P. M., an indication in any disease.

Dose: It is generally admitted that this remedy acts only in the higher potencies, the 30th being best.

Magnesia phosphorica.

(Phosphate of magnesia. Triturated with sugar of milk.)

One of the tissue remedies.

Magnesia phos. is the *pain* remedy where pain is sharp or acute. Headache, faceache, toothache, stomachache, neuralgia, menstrual colic, nerve pains, colors before the eyes, or spots; loss of smell.

Angina pectoris.

Cramps and spasms, whooping cough, cramps of muscles, tetanus, twitching, hiccough, St. Vitus' dance, chorea, spasmodic retention of urine, spasmodic cough, trembling, alcoholism, writer's cramp, hysteria, intense itching, heart pain, asthma.

Enlarged prostate, hæmorrhoids, constipation. Running watery colds, worse from cold, relieved by warmth.

Tongue, as a rule, is clean.

Dose: 3x to 12x trituration.

Melilotus.

(Yellow melilot. Tincture from the fresh flowers.)

Intensely *red face* and profuse *nosebleed, congestion,* point to this remedy.

It is said that if any one has "a headache, pain in the chest, somach or anywhere else," this remedy will relieve it in five minutes.

Furious *neuralgic headaches.*

Where there is, or was, great *hæmorrhage,* this remedy gives relief—in such cases the face may be deathly pale.

Mania, *delirium tremens.*

Dose: 1x to 3d potency. (Whether the *Melilotus off.* or *Melilotus alb.* acts better is an open question. It is generally believed that there is little if any difference between them.)

Mercurius vivus.

(Pure mercury triturated with sugar of milk.)

A *moist, flabby tongue, moist mouth, spongy gums,* and a *bad breath* indicate this remedy.

Profuse, oily, strong smelling sweat which does not relieve indicate it in rheumatism, bronchitis, pneumonia or any other disease.

Coughs, with above indications, *slimy,* ropy, nasty, coryza, night sweats.

Sore throat with constant desire to swallow the saliva though swallowing is painful.

Quinsy.

Vertigo when lying down.

The skin is nearly always *moist* when this remedy is indicated.

Syphilis, the chief remedy.

Diarrhœa with much painful straining.

Liver disease, inflammation, jaundice.

Sneezing, running at the nose, which is red and sore. Eyelids red, thick and swollen. "Colds."

Worse at night, from warm room and warm bed.

Dose: 6x to 30th potency.

Mercurius corrosivus.

(Corrosive sublimate. Trituration and dilutions.)

In *dysentery, bloody flux,* with constant *pain-*

ful straining. Autumnal dysentery. Pain in rectum.

Gonorrhœa, second stage, greenish discharge.

Severe *burning* soreness of the eyes, ophthalmia, photophobia; excoriating tears. Syphilitic iritis.

Very violent coryza with very sore, burning nostrils.

Dose: 6th to 30th potency.

Mercurius dulcis.

(Calomel. Triturated with sugar of milk.)

It affects chiefly the *oral mucosa, liver and small intestines;* the *skin is flabby* and ill nourished. Eustachian catarrh with deafness and tinnitus aurium. Diarrhœa with soreness of anus.

Prostatitis.

Dose: 3d to 6th trituration.

Mercurius jodatus flavus.

(Yellow iodide of mercury. Triturated with sugar of milk.)

This is indicated in common forms of *sore throat,* with pronounced tendency to glandular

enlargements. Small ulcers in the fauces; patches in the throat. Worse on right side.
Syphilis.
Dose: 3x trituration.

Mercurius jodatus ruber.

(Red iodide of mercury. Triturated with sugar of milk.)

Ulcerated sore throat, especially on left side, with much glandular swelling.
Diphtheria.
Dose: 3d trituration.

Mezereum.

(Spurge olive. Tincture from fresh bark.)

Pain in the *bones*, syphilitic bone pains.

Itching eruptions on the body; *intolerable itching*, compelling scratching until blood comes. *Eczema.* Shingles.

Neuralgia, worse from eating, alleviated by heat; connected with decayed teeth.

Eruptions around the mouth.

Dose: 3d to 30th potency.

Millefolium.

(Yarrow. Tincture of whole fresh plant.)

Useful in various types of hæmorrhage; chiefly florid. Bad effects from a fall from a height, sprains.

Dose: Tincture to third potency is used.

Moschus.

(Musk. Tincture from whole bag.)

The chief sphere of this drug is in *hysteria* and *nervous palpitation*.

Faints easily.

Suppressed menses, choking in throat, sudden dyspnœa, oppression in chest.

Spasmodic *nervous hiccough*.

Dose: 1st to 6th potency.

Natrum muriaticum.

(Common salt. One part by weight dissolved in nine parts by weight of distilled water, succeeding potencies run up with alcohol or prepared by trituration.)

(No drug in the homœopathic Materia Medica better illustrates the power of "potencies" than does this one which in its crude state we eat with food every day. The "Austrian provers" doubted the pathogenesis of Hahnemann and made a thorough reproving and were compelled to admit that in its potentized form it is a powerful drug.)

Despairing, helpless feeling; emaciation; con-

stant thirst; dry mouth; constipation, marks this drug.

Anæmia, pale face, headache, palpitation, depressed, yet patient eats well. Thin, scrawny neck.

Chronic *headache* in the anæmic. Headaches of pale school children.

Lips dry and *corners of mouth* sore.

Deep cracks in middle of upper or lower lip.

"Fever blisters." Clear, frothy mucus.

Abnormal craving for salt.

"Hangnails."

Tetter at bend of joints crack, crust and ooze.

Intermittent fever. Chill about 10 or 11 A. M.; thirst before and during chill, but none in fever; intense headache. Intermittents that have been suppressed but not cured with quinine.

Coryza, with clear droppings of mucus like clear water.

Ailments *worse at the seashore.*

Marasmus, neck much emaciated, yet child *eats ravenously;* anal fissure.

Scorbutic gums, dry mouth, mapped tongue.

Vagina dry and sore.

Backache, back feels broken.

Greasy skin.

White, frothy saliva.

Dose: 30th to 200th potency.

Natrum phosphoricum.

(Phosphate of soda. Triturated with sugar of milk.)

One of the "tissue" remedies.

The keynotes of *Natrum phos.* in general are *acidity and sourness.* Sour, acid eructations and vomiting.

Gout and rheumatism of the joints. Sour smelling sweat, or acid. Uric acid.

Yellow secretions in the eyes. Catarrhal conditions, with *yellow,* excoriating discharges. Catarrh of the bladder.

Intermittent fever, with sour, acid vomiting.

Spermatorrhœa, weak back, debilitated.

Acid diarrhœa. "Acid children," vomit sour matter.

Swollen sebaceous glands. Gonorrhœa.

Heartburn, waterbrash, gastric acidity. Acid dyspepsia.

Dose: 3x to 12x trituration.

Natrum sulphuricum.

(Sodium sulphate. Triturated with sugar of milk.)

Natrum sulph. is a *bilious bitter* remedy. *Bilious* fever. *Bilious,* bitter vomiting, or eructations, or diarrhœa. Sick headache. *Bitter taste.* Brown tongue.

Influenza. *Grippe,* usually the only remedy needed.

Complaints worse from wet weather is a strong feature.

Jaundice. Yellow fever. Flatulent colic. Fever and ague. Liver diseases.

Catarrh, with greenish-yellow discharges.

Diabetes and kidney diseases.

Dyspepsia.

Asthma and bronchial catarrh, with yellow, greenish expectoration.

Worse from dampness.

Dose: 3x to 12x trituration.

Nitricum acidum.

(Nitric acid. One part by weight dissolved in nine parts by weight of distilled water constitutes the 1st decimal potency.)

Outlets of body, mouth, anus, nose, etc., *cracked, fissured, sore,* ulcerated or scabby. Ulcerated, spongy gums. Pains, in any part, seem as from a splinter.

Great pain in anus *after stool.*

Clears up cases of syphilis that have been overdrugged by the old school treatment. Syphilitic iritis.

Sore throat as from splinters in it.

Dose: 3d to 30th potency.

Nux moschata.

(Nutmeg. Tincture from powdered nuts.)

The sphere of this drug is chiefly *mental*. *Loss of memory.* Vanishing thoughts. Absent minded. *Stupor.* Fainting spells. Hysteria. Coma. *Sleepiness with all complaints. Very dry mouth.*

Flatulence, everything seems to turn to wind. Cholera infantum.

Nervous aphonia. Sleeping sickness.

Children who, while unusually bright, nevertheless seem unable to learn to talk.

Dose: 6th, 30th and 200th potencies.

Nux vomica.

(Poison nut. Tincture from powdered nuts.)

Hypersensitive. Chilliness. Twitching.

One great use of this great remedy is to administer it (30th potency) to patients coming from old school hands who have been *over-drugged,* have been high livers, taken much patent medicine, aromatics, spices or have been long under allopathic treatment.

Nux vomica will work wonders in such cases.

Suitable to the ills of those who lead a *sedentary life.* Constipation, frequent desire, but passes little or nothing.

For the ills of heavy *liquor drinkers*.
Frontal headache, vertigo.
Angry, irritable.
Awakes every morning about 3 or 4 o'clock and unable to go to sleep again.
Feels worse after awakening. Hot, red face.
Stuffy colds, stopped up, little or no discharge.
Liver disease brought on by alcoholic drinks.
Hernia, rupture; it has won green laurels here.
Dose: θ to 30th potency.

Œnanthe crocata.

(Water hemlock. Tincture from the fresh root.)

The chief use of this remedy is in *epilepsy; violent convulsions; opisthotonos;* facial twitchings; foaming at mouth. Has cured many cases.
Dose: 1x to 6th potency.

Opium.

(Tincture from dry powdered opium.)

A dark and red face; stertorous breathing; torpor; depression; drowsiness; besotted appearance, eyes half closed; call for this drug.
Apoplexy, stupor, cool extremities.
Cerebral hæmorrhage.
Paralysis, recent.

Obstinate constipation, violent colic. *Lead* colic. Fæcal vomiting.

Complaints preceded by somnolence and followed by wakefulness.

Dose: 3d to 30th potency.

Passiflora incarnata.

(Passion flower. Tincture from fresh flowering plant.)

An unproved drug, an anti-spasmodic and while not a narcotic produces quiet sleep.

Has been successfully used in insomnia of nervous neuralgia, nervousness, irregular pains of pregnancy, dysmenorrhœa, morphine habit, tetanus, and many other diseases; in short, it is indicated wherever the bromides, chloral, morphine, etc., are indicated and will give better results.

Dose: From five drops to a teaspoonful of the θ, or five mother tincture tablets.

Petroleum.

(Rock oil. One part by weight of the Rangoon oil dissolved in 99 parts by weight of alcohol.)

Eczema that is worse in winter and goes away in summer.

Hands, lips, fingers and nose crack open and bleed. *Finger tips* cracked and raw. Raw eruptions.

Foul smell from *sweat of armpits* and *feet*. Feet tender.

Rheumatism where there is *cracking of joints*.

Raw margins of *eyelids*.

Cold feeling in the heart.

Dose: 3d to 6th potency.

Phosphoric acid.

(One part by weight of purified glacial phosphoric acid dissolved in ninety parts by weight of distilled water and then add ten parts of alcohol.)

Profuse colorless urine, *diabetes*.

Debility from excessive *coition, masturbation* or *seminal emissions*, weak, dizzy, despairing. *Impotence*.

For the ills of the young who *grow too fast,* study too hard; *headache*. "Growing pains."

Painless, profuse diarrhœa.

Typhoid fever, with quiet delirium and stupor, yet when aroused patient is conscious.

Dose: 1st to 3d potency.

Phosphorus.

(Saturated alcoholic solution.)

Burning pains, fatty degeneration, caries, exhaustion, prostration, mental exertion dreaded, oppression of chest, little thirst and weak legs,

little fever, characterize this dangerous drug. *Worse when lying on left side.*
Small wounds bleed freely. Hæmorrhagic diathesis. Cancerous ulcerations, or sores, *bleeding freely. Easy bleeding.*
Softening of the brain, vertigo, tired. Brain feels tired. Heavy pressure on top of head.
Threatened cataract; things appear in a gray mist.
Bleeding, nasal polypi.
Necrosis or *caries* of bones.
As soon as *cold water* becomes *warm* in the stomach it is *vomited*. Burning fermentation in the stomach.
Malignant jaundice. Cirrhosis of liver.
Chronic, *painless* diarrhœa.
Laryngitis, with aphonia, chronic cough.
Easy hæmorrhage from the lungs, *pneumonia*, no fever, great oppression on the chest.
Phthisis, bright red blood, sweet or salty tasting expectoration.
Fatty degeneration of the heart.
Spinal irritation; burning pain.
Locomotor ataxia. *Heat running up the back.*
Fungous bleeding excrescences.
Vomiting of coffee-ground looking matter.
Ulcers of stomach. *Hungry*, eating relieves but soon hungry again.

Doesn't want to be alone; afraid in the dark.

The typical *Phosphorus* patient is slender, fair, waxy-faced, with dark rings about the eyes.

Dose: 6th to 30th, or 200th potency, and do not give it oftener than once a day.

Phytolacca decandra.

(Poke root. Tincture from the fresh roots.)

Sore throat, red and inflamed, white spots; high fever, *intense aching* of head, back and limbs calls for this remedy. Non-malignant diphtheria, tonsillitis, scarlatina or pharyngitis, *bluish tonsils;* syphilitic bone pains or rheumatism.

Burning in throat.

Wants to bite teeth together or gums; *dentition.*

Caked breasts, breasts hard, swollen and painful; tumors on breasts, nipples sore and cracked.

(Use also *Phytolacca cerate* in this condition.)

Dose: 1x, 3d to 30th potency.

Picric acid.

(One part by weight dissolved in ninety-nine parts by weight of alcohol.)

Neurasthenia and *brain-fag;* disintegrates the red blood corpuscles; degeneration of spinal cord; pernicious anæmia.

Intense *sexual excitement, priapism,* profound exhaustion.

Very heavy, weary, tired feeling of entire body.

Dose: 3d potency to 30th, the latter preferable.

Plantago.

(Plantain. Tincture of the whole fresh plant.)

Good in earache, toothache and neuralgia when patient is sensitive to touch and cold air.

Dose: Mother tincture and lower potencies. It is also used locally with good effect.

Platina.

(Precipitated metal. Triturated with sugar of milk.)

Its sphere is *sexual, nervous and mental;* exalts self and has contempt for others. Numbness and coldness are characteristic. Chiefly indicated in women.

Nymphomania, puerperal nymphomania, excessive sexual desire in young girls, *hysteria.* Young boys almost imbecile from *excessive masturbation, satyriasis.*

Constipation caused by traveling.

Dose: 3d to 30th potency.

Plumbum metallicum.

(Lead. Precipitated metal triturated with sugar of milk.)

Paralysis, constipation, colic, griping spasms, emaciation, hardening of tissue, apathy and *palsy* point to this drug.

Abdomen seems as if *drawn back to spine,* impacted fæces, violent pains about the *navel,* navel seems pulled backward. *Spinal paralysis, complete paralysis of limbs,* wrist drop of paralysis, *paralytic conditions* generally.

Spasmodic drawing in of anus.

Chlorosis, with inveterate constipation.

Generally dry skin.

Dose: 6th to 30th potency.

Podophyllum.

(Mandrake. May apple. Tincture of the fresh root.)

It affects chiefly the duodenum, liver and rectum. Adapted to the bilious temperament.

It is indicated in diarrhœa, cholera infantum, cholera morbus and is serviceable in bilious states generally with gastro-intestinal symptoms.

Special indications are aggravation in the morning, worse in hot weather, and tendency to anal prolapsus.

Dose: Tincture to the sixth potency may be used.

Pulsatilla.

(Wind flower. Tincture from the whole flowering plant.)

The classical *Pulsatilla* patient is a female, blonde, gentle and tearful; thirstless; *worse in warm room, better in the open air,* yet chilly; discharges bland, thick and greenish yellow; wandering, shifting pains, yet there are many males who also need this polychrest at times.

Indigestion; bad bitter taste; indigestion from fat or rich food. *Loss of taste.* Furred *tongue.*

Conjunctivitis; ophthalmia; profuse, thick, bland discharge. *Styes* on the eyes.

Earache. Discharge of thick pus from the ears.

Nasal catarrh, profuse, thick, non-excoriating discharge.

Neuralgia *worse from warmth,* better in open air.

Orchitis. Neuralgia of testicles.

Menses late, scanty or suppressed.

Menstrual troubles *from getting wet.* Painful menstruation. Menstrual troubles of *blondes. Chlorosis.*

Varicose veins.

Relief in cool, open air or from cold applications are the red letter symptoms of this drug.

Thirstlessness, yet dry mouth.

Especially indicated where there has been an over-drugging of *iron* and *quinine*.
Dose: 6th to 30th potency.

Pyrogenium.

(Rotten, lean meat. Tincture from same.)

This is an almost unproved remedy introduced by Dr. J. Compton Burnett, who found it wonderfully curative in all typhoid and septic fevers. The chief indication by Burnett is the diagnosis of "typhoid."
Dose: 6th to 30th potency.

Ranunculus bulbosus.

(Buttercup. Tincture of the entire fresh plant.)

It acts especially on the muscular tissue and skin, and its effect on the chest walls is characteristic. Pleurodynia. Intercostal rheumatism. Neuralgia. Pains are worse from motion.

Soreness in the chest, rheumatic pains, stitches.
Dose: First to third dilution may be used.

Ratanhia.

(Krameria. Tincture from dried root.)

This remedy is peculiarly an anal one—*itching* of anus, anal *fissure* and *hæmorrhoids* that burn

like fire. Anus burns long after stools. It is given internally and applied externally in form of suppositories or cerate.
Dose: 3d to 6th potency.

Rheum.

(Rhubarb. Tincture of the dried root.)

It is useful in diarrhœa with distinctly sour smell, and teething troubles. The child smells sour. Much saliva, restless, irritable.

Particularly suited to infants and children as well as pregnant and nursing women.

Dose: The third to the sixth potency is used.

Rhus toxicodendron.

(Poison oak. Tincture from the fresh leaves.)

Worse when quiet is a marked characteristic of this drug; pain drives patient to motion and he feels better after moving about; is lame and stiff when starting, but with motion this is relieved. Continual change of position. Effect of *sprains or strains;* also from getting wet. Ills worse from wet, damp weather, as rheumatic pains between the shoulders, etc.

Raw, granulated eyelids.

Erysipelas, when vesicles form. Herpes. *Eczema. Itching, burning,* are its keynotes in skin diseases.

Headache worse from touch.

Rheumatism. Lumbago. Especially from exposure to wet. Colds from getting wet. Glands swollen from getting wet.

In typhoid where there is a *red triangular patch* on the tip of the tongue.

Small-pox, black pustules.

Rhus patient is worse in wet or cold wet weather and better in dry warmth, from stretching and rubbing. A great rheumatic remedy.

Dose: 6th to 30th potency.

Rumex.

(Yellow dock. Tincture of the fresh root.)

Cough caused by constant tickling sensation in the pit of the throat; aggravated by touching the throat and by inhaling cold air. Larynx is very sensitive. Used in the early stages of whooping cough; night cough of phthisis. Cough preventing sleep.

Dose: The third to the sixth potency is used.

Ruta graveolens.

(Rue. Tincture from fresh plant before blooming.)

Over-strained eyes; headache; feel weary, vision dim, ache as if strained; burn. *Neuralgia* in eyes.

Prolapsus of rectum.

Pains in bones, joints and cartilages as if bruised, tendency to deposits. Pains, rheumatism, in wrists or ankles. Lameness after sprains. Dose: 3d to 6th potency. Peculiar modality of being worse from lying down.

Sabadilla.

(Indian caustic barley. Tincture from powdered seeds.)

Relief in the open air, yet sensitive to cold.

Useful in *imaginary disease,* where patient imagines so and so ails him when it does not.

Influenza, with violent sneezing, lachrymation, watery discharge, itching, tingling in the nose. *Hay fever. Grippe.*

Chills beginning in the extremities and running up the body.

Wants warm food and drink.

Dose: 3d to 30th potency.

Sanguinaria Canadensis.

(Blood root. Tincture of fresh root.)

Sick headache, pain begins in back of head, or occiput, settles over right eye; patient wants to be in a dark room, perfectly quiet and no odors. Headache that increases as the sun rises and decreases as it goes down.

Rush of blood to the head, veins distended.

Burning sensation. Better lying down, vomiting of bile.

Dose: 1x to 6th potency.

Secale cornutum.

(Ergot. Tincture of the fresh spurs.)

Useful when there is a contraction of the unstriped muscular fibres. Contraction and relaxation alternately.

Anæmic conditions, coldness, numbness, petechiæ, mortification, gangrene, dry gangrene. Face pinched and sunken.

Skin dry, shriveled and brittle.

All symptoms are worse from external heat.

Uterine hæmorrhages; passive, painless flow of dark, thin blood.

Dose: Tincture to 30th potency.

Senecio aureus.

(Ragwort. Tincture from fresh blooming plant.)

Trembling; nervous; *menses retarded* or *suppressed; dysmenorrhœa.*

Backache. Uterine irritation or prolapse.

May be regarded as a "uterine tonic" when there is an atonic condition of uterus or ovaries; strengthens functional activities, and aids digestion in such cases. May be classed among the empiric remedies and is reputed to be low in action.

Dose: 1x to 6th potency.

Sepia.

(Dried inky juice of cuttle-fish. Tincture prepared from powdered sepia.)

Acts on portal system; venous congestion. Bearing down sensation in women; apt to be chilly. Its sphere is largely in abdomen and pelvis of women.

Yellow saddle across the nose, *yellow* spots on face, liver spots, general *yellowness,* especially in women, strongly indicate this remedy. *Dark rings* about the eyes. Headache from uterine causes in this class of women. Flushes of heat. Foul sweat. Easily fatigued. *Leucorrhœa,* yellow or greenish, itching. Weak back.

Dyspepsia; goneness of stomach; faintness, emptiness; craves pickles or sour things. Liver feels sore, brown spots on body.

Scaly eruptions on the legs.

Chronic nasal catarrh.

Facial neuralgia of pregnancy.

Herpes. Acne. Eruption around the joints. Chronic gleet.

Dose: 6th to 30th potency.

Silicea.

(Pure precipitated silicea. Triturated with sugar of milk.)

A *constitutional* remedy; imperfectly nourished, but *not* for want of food.

Suppuration—carbuncles, whitlow, ulcers, fistules, boils, vaccination sores, cancer; all inflammation ending in watery suppuration.

Head sweat in children; big belly, but small limbs, old looking.

Constipation; stool protrudes and then slips back.

Lack of vital force and heat; takes cold easily; wraps up head; very sensitive to cold or even cool air. *Chronic headache.*

Unhealthy, ill smelling *foot sweat.*

Bone diseases, caries, hip joint disease.

Hectic fever; night sweats; phthisis.

Dose: 6th to 30th potency. Acts better in higher potency.

Spigelia.

(Pink root. Tincture from dried plant.)

Intense pain characterizes this remedy.

Neuralgia; pain in the eyes; neuralgic headaches.

Also the most *violent palpitation of the heart,*

so violent as to be visible. *Carditis.* Neuralgia of the heart.

Rheumatism, as if sprained in the joints.

Neuralgic toothache.

Dose: Tincture to 30th potency. May claim that the tincture acts better in neuralgia than the potency.

Spongia.

(Tincture from roasted Turkish sponges.)

The chief use of this remedy is in the treatment of *croup,* where it follows well after *Aconite.* It is especially indicated when the cough is harsh and dry, *sounding like a saw being driven through a board.* Also when patient awakes from sleep with a paroxysm of coughing, in croup.

Chronic hoarseness.

Dose: 3d to 30th potency.

Stannum.

(Tin. Trituration of the precipitated metal with sugar of milk.)

Weakness is the keynote of this drug. Weak chest, repugnance to talking. Talking tires the patient. Descending stairs tires patient.

Chronic catarrh; hawks up much lumpy mucus with sweetish taste,

Phthisis, with much expectoration, greenish and sweetish or salty taste.

Causes lumbrici and ascarides to pass in large quantities if they be present (6x trit.).

Marked *weakness* must be present to indicate this remedy, and the patient is generally sad and despondent.

Dose: 6x to 15x potency.

Staphisagria.

(Stavesacre. Tincture from ripe seed.)

Very irritable, takes offense at trifles. Pale face, sunken eyes, blue rings about them. Effects of masturbation.

Teeth turn black and decay early.

Dry, itching eruptions.

Cauliflower excrescences. Nodosities, styes.

Where child is persistently *lousy* this remedy is indicated, *internally.* It also has a place with *Chamomilla* in the treatment of cross, petulant children, though the latter remedy seems more proper for the peevishness of children who suffer actual physical discomfort.

Dose: 3d to 30th potency.

Sticta pulmonaria.

(Lungwort. Tincture of the fresh lichen.)

Coryza, bronchial catarrh and influenza when

there is dryness of the mucous membrane, with nervous and rheumatic symptoms. There is pain, heaviness and pressure in forehead, dullness, and at root of nose, so often felt in coryzas, but there is no running from the nose or watery eyes. It is for "dry colds." Also for hay fever with these characteristics.

Hard, dry, barking, almost croupy cough; worse at night with little or no expectoration.

Dose: Tincture to 6th potency is used.

Stramonium.

(Thorn apple. Tincture from the fresh plant in flower and fruit.)

The chief guide to this drug is *delirium*. Wild mania, sees things springing at him; hears voices, spirits talking to him; very loquacious; talks foolishly; fears to be in the dark or alone; has all sorts of queer fancies. Religious mania Ridiculous scruples.

Fear of water.

All motions hasty—startling—spasmodic.

Vertigo in the dark.

Stuttering, stammering.

Dribbling urine.

Nymphomania preceding menstruation.

Very little pain in *Stramonium* cases.

Dose: 3d to 30th potency.

Sulphur.

(Brimstone. Washed sublimed sulphur triturated with sugar of milk. Also prepared as a tincture.)

This is Hahnemann's greatest "antipsoric," and there are few diseases in which it may not come into play.

One indication is that: "When seemingly well indicated drugs do not act" then give *Sulphur*—it is the psora, or hereditary underlying the more superficial disease, that is in the way.

Burning is a great indication—burning eyes, on top of the head, rectum, soles of feet—anywhere. Also *flushes of heat*. All *orifices* of body are apt to be *red*.

The *Sulphur* patient has a decided aversion to washing. Dirty looking skin, harsh and dry; dry hair; eczema, acne, dry porrigo, all manner of skin diseases.

Many cases of general ill health rapidly clear up under *Sulphur*.

Rheumatism and chronic lumbago; diarrhœa.

In later stages of pneumonia and pleurisy.

Neuralgia.

Fever, day after day, with no sweat.

Scrofula. Marasmus. Nearly always hungry. Chronic catarrh, scabby nose.

Hot head and cold feet, or *vice versa.*

Itch, give internally, while killing the itch mites with proper applications.

Engorged liver. Hæmorrhoids, constipation. Burning leucorrhœa.

Dose: 1x to 30th potency—the latter the better.

Tabacum.

(Tobacco. Tincture of dry leaves from Havana.)

Relaxation and paralysis of the involuntary muscular system. Præcordial oppression, nausea, vertigo, cold sweat, debility. Often indicated and very useful in sea-sickness.

Dose: The 3d to 30th and even higher potencies are used.

Tarantula Cubensis.

(Cuban spider. Tincture from the entire living spider.)

Malignant, deep-reaching carbuncles, exceedingly painful; purplish color. Abscesses, felons. Ulceration presenting the characteristic *malignant purplish hue and pain*.

Malignant diphtheria, onset sudden and violent.

Dose: 6th to 30th potency.

Terebinthina.

(Turpentine. One part by weight of purified oil of turpentine to ninety-nine parts by weight of alcohol.)

Inflammation of the kidneys, strangury.

Bloody urine, or it becomes dark and smoky with blood in it. It is an anti-hæmorrhagic remedy.
Tympanitis, especially in typhoid.
Very painful in region of the kidneys; inflammation.
Dysuria, or urine suppressed. Urethritis with painful erections.
Dose: 1st to 6th potency.

Thlaspi bursa pastoris.

(Shepherd's purse. Tincture from fresh flowering plant.)

This may be called a Rademacher remedy. He gave it in thirty-drop doses of the tincture to clear from the kidneys "brick dust," uric acid and calculus. It has also been used in hæmorrhages from the kidneys. Also bladder troubles of old men.

Dose: One to twenty drops of θ in water.

Thuja.

(Arbor Vitæ. Tincture from the fresh leaves.)

This is Hahnemann's great "anti-sycotic" remedy. *Excrescences under beard or hair; condylomata, polypi, fig warts; gonorrhœa* and its remote effects, especially if it had been suppressed; *gleet. Gonorrhœal rheumatism.*

Burnett used it very extensively for what he termed "vaccinosis," *i. e.*, the chronic ill health from which thousands suffer that, unknowingly, is implanted by vaccination. He prescribed the 30th potency, for all who have "not been as well" since vaccination. He had some wonderful results from this remedy.

Bœnninghausen regarded it as a sure prophylactic against small-pox; also a remedy as soon as the vesicles had filled to promote desiccation and prevent scars.

Like *Sulphur* it is often needed as an intercurrent remedy in the sycotic diathesis as *Sulphur* is in the psoric.

Dose: θ to 30th (the latter preferable).

Urtica urens.

(Common nettle. Tincture from entire flowering plant.)

Highly commended by Burnett in five-drop doses of the θ for *gout*.

Nettle rash, hives, urticaria.

Dose: θ to 3x potency.

Ustilago.

(Corn-smut. Tincture or trituration.)

Bright, partly clotted hæmorrhages from passive congestion of uterus; especially at climacteric. Excessive menstruation.

Dose: The tincture to the third potency is used.

Veratrum album.

(White hellebore. Tincture from dried roots.)

Cramps, cold sweat, watery *diarrhœa* and *vomiting, pain,* prostration and collapse point to this remedy.

Asiatic cholera, rice water discharges.

Any acute state with *cold sweat on forehead.*

Watery diarrhœa with great pain, "bellyache."

Dose: 3d to 30th potency.

Veratrum viride.

(Swamp hellebore. Tincture from fresh roots.)

Dr. E. B. Nash in his *Leaders in Homœopathic Therapeutics* says of this remedy that when it was in its hey-day in the treatment of pneumonia: "One day I left a patient, relieved by this remedy, of an acute and violent attack of pneumonia, to go to a town five miles distant, and when I returned found my patient dead. Then I watched others treated with this remedy and found every little while a patient with pneumonia dropping out *suddenly* when they were reported better." "It is not desirable (it is wrong) to control or *depress the pulse* regardless of all other conditions." "The patients, who had weak hearts, were killed by this powerful heart depressant. A quickened circulation is salutary in all inflammatory diseases." "Next to *Digitalis, Veratrum viride* slows the pulse, as is abundantly shown in its provings."

Homœopathically, it would be indicated in a very slow pulse.

Dose: 6th to 30th potency.

Zincum metallicum.

(Metallic zinc. The pure metal triturated with sugar of milk.)

It has been said "what iron is to the blood, zinc is to the nerves."

Trembling all over, is a marked leader to this drug.

Paralysis.

Brain diseases. Child bores its head into the pillow, or rolls it from side to side.

Unable to expectorate, yet expectoration relieves. General paresis.

Hydrocephalus.

Meningitis following suppressed exanthema. Sciatica, with restless feet.

Spinal irritation.

Neuralgia of elbow joints.

Always worse from alcoholic stimulants.

Trembling and "the fidgets" are great leaders in this powerful remedy.

Dose: 6th to 30th potency.

INDEX.

Abscess, 44
Abrotanum, 120
Acne, 44
Aconite, 120
Æsculus hip., 121
Addison's disease, 44
Agaricus mus., 122
Agnus castus, 122
Alcoholism, 44
Aletris far., 122
Allium cepa, 123
Aloe, 123
Alum, 124
Alumen, 124
Alumina, 124
Amaurosis, 45
Ambergris, 124
Ambra grisea, 124
Amenorrhœa, 45
American hemp, 145
Ammonium carb., 125
Anacardium orient., 125
Anæmia, 45
Angina pectoris, 45
Antimonium crudum, 126
Antimonium tartaricum,
Apis mel., 127
Aphthæ, 46
Apocynum cannabinum, 128
Apoplexy, 46
Appendicitis, 47
Arbor vitæ, 212

Argentum met., 129
Argentum nit., 130
Arnica montana, 130
Arsenicum album, 131
Arsenious acid, 131
Arthritis, 47
Arundo Mauritianica, 133
Asafœtida, 134
Asthma, 48
Attenuations, 33
Aurum met., 133
Arum tryphillum, 132

Bacillinum, 134
Backache, 49
Baptisia, 135
Barberry, 138
Baryta carb., 136
Bean of St. Ignatius, 172
Beech drop, 163
Belladonna, 136
Benzoic acid, 137
Berberis vul., 138
Bichromate of potash, 175
Bismuthum, 138
Bitter sweet, 162
Black and blue, 73
Black lead, 167
Black snake root, 153
Bladder, 50
Blue cohosh, 148
Bilious attack, 50
Blue flag, 174
Blue gum tree, 163

INDEX.

Blood poisoning, 51
Bloodroot, 203
Boils, 52
Bones, 52
Boneset, 164
Books, Homœopathic, 23
Borax, 138
Brain, 53
Bronchitis, 53
Bruises, 53
Bryonia, 139
Buttercup, 200

Cactus grandiflorus, 140
Caladium seg., 141
Calcium sulphide (impure), 170
Calcarea carbonica, 141
Calcarea fluorica, 142
Calcarea phosphorica, 143
Calendula, 144
Calculus, 54
Camphora, 145
Canadian hemp., 128
Cancer, 54
Cannabis Indica, 145
Cannabis sativa, 146
Cantharis, 147
Capsicum, 147
Carbonate of barium, 136
Carbo vegetabilis, 147
Carbuncle, 55
Carduus Marianus, 148
Catalepsy, 56
Cataract, 56
Catarrh, 56
Caulophyllum, 148
Causticum, 149
Cedron, 150
Cerebro-spinal meningitis, 89
Chamomilla, 150
Charcoal, 147

Chaste tree, 122
Chelidonium maus, 157
Chest, 57
Chicken-pox, 57
Chilblain, 58
Chills and fever, 87
Chimaphilla umbellata, 152
Chininum ars., 152
China, 154
Cholera Asiatica, 58
Cholera infantum, 59
Cholera morbus, 60
Chorea, 60
"Chronic Diseases, The," 18
Cicuta virosa, 152
Cimicifuga racemosa, 157
Cina, 153
Cinchona, 154
Cocculus Indicus, 154
Clematis erecta, 155
Club moss, 181
Coccus cacti, 155
Coffea cruda, 156
Colds, 56, 60
Colic, 60
Colchicum, 156
Collinsonia Can., 157
Colocynth, 157
Cone flower, Purple, 162
Conium mac., 157
Consumption, 62
Convulsions, 63
Cough, 64
Constipation, 61
Corrosive sublimate, 184
Copper, 160
Corallium rubrum, 158
Cramps, 66
Croup, 66
Crocus sativa, 159
Crotalus horridus, 159

INDEX. 219

Croton tiglium, 160
Cuban spider, 211
Cucumber, bitter, 157
Cuprum met., 160

Debility, 67
Dentition, 67
Diabetes, 67
Diarrhœa, 68
Digitalis, 161
Dilutions, 33
Dioscorea vil., 161
Diphtheria, 69
Disks, 9
Dispensing, 36
Dose, Pellets, 117
Dosage and Potency, 14
Dropsy, 69
Drosera rotund., 161
Drug Proving, 12
Dulcamara, 162
Dysentery, 70
Dyspepsia, 71

Ear, 72
Echinacea, 162
Ecchymosis, 73
Eczema, 73
Emissions, seminal, 74
Epilepsy, 74
Epiphegus, 163
Ergot, 204
Erigeron, 163
Erysipelas, 75
Eucalyptus, 163
Eupatorium per., 164
Euphrasia, 164
Eyebright, 164
Eyes, 75

Feet, 76
Ferrum phos., 165
Ferrum met., 165

Fever, 81
Flea bane, 163
Fluorspar, 142
Fool's parsley, 116
Fox glove, 161

Gangrene, 77
Gastralgia, 77
Gelsemium, 166
Glandular swelling, 77
Glonoine, 67
Goitre, 78
Gold, 123
Golden seal, 171
Gonorrhœa, 78
Gout, 47, 79
Graphites, 167
Grippe, 86

Hæmorrhage, 80
Hæmorrhoids, 80
Hahnemann, 9
Hamamelis Virginica, 108
Hands, 81
Hashish, 145
Hay fever, 81
Headache, 82
Heart, 83
Hellebore, swamp, 214
Hellebore, white, 214
Helleborus niger, 169
Helonias dioica, 169
Hemlock poison, 157
Henbane, 171
Hepar sulphur. calcareum, 170
Hernia, 84
Hiccough, 84
Hoarseness, 84
Honey bee, 127
Homœopathic books, 23

INDEX

Homœopathic medicines, 30
"Homœopathic Vaccination," 107
Horse-chestnut, 121
"How do your medicines act?" 38
Hydrastis Canadensis, 171
Hydrocephalus, 84
Hydrophobia, 85
Hyoscyamus, 171
Hypericum perforatum, 172
Hysteria, 85

"I want the latest," 13
Ignatia, 172
Indian caustic barley, 203
Indian hemp, 128
Indian tobacco, 181
Indian turnip, 132
Influenza, 86
Intermittent fever, 87
Insomnia, 106
Iodium, 173
Ipecacuanha, 173
Irritation, 88
Iris versicolor, 174
Iron, 165

Jaundice, 88
Jessamine, 166

Kali bichromicum, 175
Kali carbonicum, 175
Kali muriaticum, 176
Kali phosphoricum, 177
Kali sulphuricum, 178
Kalmia latifolia, 178
Kidneys, 89
Krameria, 200

Kreosotum, 179

Lachesis, 179
Laurel, mountain, 179
Laryngitis, 89
Lead, 198
Lead, black, 167
Ledum palustre, 180
Leptandra, 180
Leucorrhœa, 90
Leopard's bane, 130
Lilium tigrinum, 181
Liver, 90
Lobelia inflata, 181
Locomotor ataxia, 91
Lumbago, 92
Lungs, 92
Lungwort, 208
Lycopodium, 181

Magnesia phosphorica, 102
Mandrake, 198
May apple, 198
Marasmus, 93
Marigold, 144
Marsh tea, 180
Meadow saffron, 156
Measles, 94
Melilotus, 183
Meningitis, 95
Menstruation, 95
Mental, 96
Mercurius corrosivus, 184
Mercurius dulcis, 185
Mercurius jod. flavus, 185
Mercurius jod. rub., 186
Mercurius vivus, 184
Mercury, 184
Mezereum, 186
Millefolium, 186

INDEX.

Monkshood, 120
Moschus, 187
Mother tinctures, 32
Mumps, 97
Mushroom, poison, 122
Musk, 187

Natrum muriaticum, 187
Natrum phosphoricum, 189
Natrum sulphuricum, 189
Nettle, 213
Neuralgia, 97
Neurasthenia, 98
Night-blooming cereus, 140
Nightshade, deadly, 136
Nitrate of silver, 130
Nitricum acidum, 190
Nitroglycerin, 167
Nose-bleed, 99
Nut, poison, 191
Nutmeg, 191
Nux moschata, 191
Nux vomica, 191

Œnanthe crocata, 192
Onion, 123
Opium, 192
Origin of Homœopathy, 10
Oyster shell, 141

Paralysis, 99
Passion flower, 193
Passiflora incarnata, 193
Peritonitis, 99
Petroleum, 193
Phosphate of iron, 165
Phosphate of lime, 143
Phosphoric acid, 194
Phosphorus, 194

Phytolacca decandra, 196
Picric acid, 196
Pink root, 206
Plantago, 197
Plantain, 197
Platina, 197
Pleurisy, 100
Pleurodynia, 100
Plumbum, 198
Pneumonia, 192
Podophyllum, 198
Poison oak, 201
Poke root, 194
Potassium chloride, 176
Potencies, 33
Prostate gland, 101
Pruritus, 88
Proving drugs, 13
Pulmonary œdema, 83
Pulsatilla, 199
Pyrogenium, 200

Quinsy, 101

Ragwort, 204
Ranunculus bulbosus, 200
Ratanhia, 200
Rattlesnake, 159
Red coral, 158
Red pepper, 147
Rectum, 101
Rheum, 201
Rheumatism, 102
Rhubarb, 201
Rhus toxicodendron, 201
Ringworm, 103
Rock oil, 193
Rue, 202
Rumex, 202
Ruta graveolens, 202

Sabadilla, 203

Saffron, 159
Saffron, meadow, 156
Salt, 187
Sanguinaria Canadensis, 200
Scarlet fever, 103
Sciatica, 104
Scrofula, 104
Secale cornutum, 204
Senecio aureus, 204
Sepia, 205
Shepherd's purse, 212
Skin, 105
Silicea, 206
Silver, 129
Sleep, 106
Small-pox, 107
Soda phosphate, 189
Sodium sulphate, 189
Southernwood, 120
Spanish fly, 146
Spermatorrhœa, 108
Spigelia, 206
Spitting of blood, 93
Spleen, 108
Spongia, 207
Spotted fever, 95
Spurge olive, 186
St. John's wort, 172
St. Mary's thistle, 148
Stannum, 207
Staphisagria, 208
Stavesacre, 208
Star grass, 122
Sticta pulmonaria, 208
Stomach, 109
Stone root, 157
Stramonium, 209
Sulphur, 210
Summer complaint, 108
Sundew, 161
Sunstroke, 108
Swellings, 44

Symptomatology, 20
Syphilis, 109

Tabacum, 211
Tablets, 17 ,
Tarantula Cubensis, 211
Tartar emetic, 127
Teeth, 110
Terebinthina, 211
Tetanus, 111
Therapeutics, 43
Thlaspi bursa pastoris, 212
Thorn apple, 208
Throat, 112
Thrush, 46
Thuja, 212
Tiger lily, 181
Tin, 207
Tincture, mother, 32
Triturations, 34
Trying Homœopathy, 37
Tuberculosis, 62
Turpentine, 211
Typhoid, 113

Unicorn, false, 169
Urinary disorders, 114
Urtica urens, 213
Ustilago, 213

Vaccinosis, 115
Vehicle for dispensing homœopathic medicines, 36
Veratrum album, 214
Veratrum viride, 214
Virgin's bower, 155
Voice, 115

Water hemlock, 192
Whooping cough, 115
Wild hops, 109